"This is a GREAT concept!"
　　　　—Dr. Bob Arnot, National TV
　　　　Medical Correspondent
　　　　New York, NY

"This is how I think. I work at McDonald's and I stay thin."
　　　　—Dawn Mott,
　　　　McDonald's Manager

"This is a truly wonderful book and is the TRUTH about maintaining a healthy and fit body."
　　　　—Dr. Marge Gibbons, Holiday, FL

"These tips are a perfectly acceptable and reasonable way to work on changing your thought process . . . this book would be effective for many people."
　　　　—Jill Zelinsky, RD, LDN
　　　　Assistant Director, Nutrition Services
　　　　The Reading Hospital, PA

"Why didn't anyone tell us this before? This is the ONLY way to stay in shape for life."
　　　　—Doreen Donovan Corkin
　　　　Mother of three, Weston, MA

How Thin People Think

How Thin People Think

464 Common Sense Tips from People Who Choose to Be Thin for Life

Written and Illustrated by
Louise A. Masano

Artes Books
NEW YORK

ISBN: 0-9759500-1-0 (e-book)
ISBN: 0-9759500-0-2 (Paperback)

This book is printed on acid-free paper.

This book reflects the views and opinions
of the author and is for entertainment purposes.
Anyone intending to lose weight should first
have consultation with a physician.

ArtesBooks
NEW YORK

www.HowThinPeopleThink.com

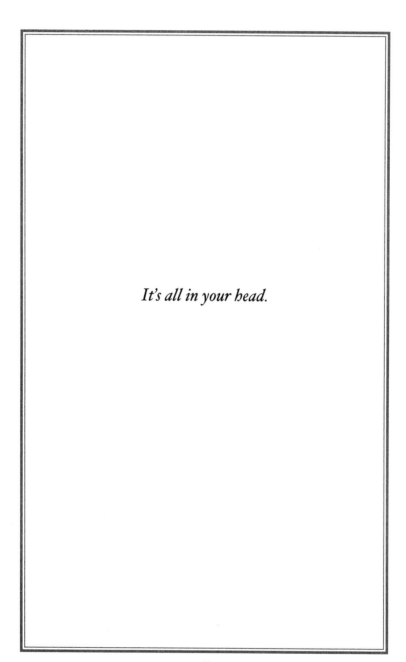

It's all in your head.

Acknowledgments

I would like to give special thanks to Tony Outhwaite, who continually encouraged me with his professional insight and his cheerleader's enthusiasm. Second to my sister Andrea, for her support and her overall aesthetic counterpoint; Dr. Carl Constein, for his initial guidance; and Kathy Antrim, my wonderful editor. Also thanks to Seton Bitterly, Erinmaura Condon, Cindy Espy, Catherine Hart, Camilla Hellman, Anna Koules, Lori Mahfouz, Heidi Masano, Kelly Masano, Dr. Kevin O'Keefe, Nancy Prall, Susan Quinn and Dr. William Sweet for their reviews; to Eric Kampmann and Gail Kump at Midpoint Books, for their commitment to this project and for being such nice people; to Ann Carole in publicity; to my Mom and Dad for their encouragement; and to all "The Thinking Thin" who have chosen to take control of their weight. They have proven to me that reasonable, daily, behavioral adjustments are the only realistic long-term solution to solving this country's weight epidemic and to enjoying a "Lifetime of Thinness."

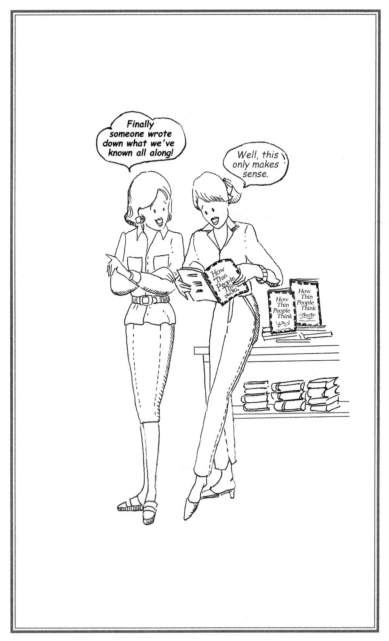

Contents

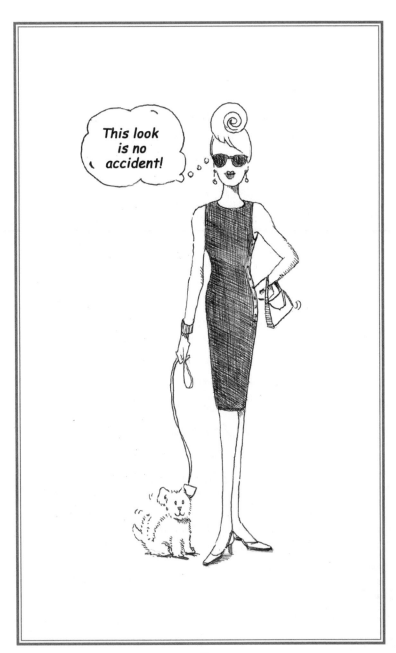

Introduction

According to U.S. government statistics,
almost 65% of Americans are overweight* —
that means close to 35% are not!

Within this 35% group are "The Thinking Thin."
(These are not the lucky ones whose metabolisms
keep them naturally slender.) They "choose" to be
thin through specific actions and attitudes, and by
having a certain mind-set about food and their bodies,
which is often different from that of those
"who are not so happy with their weight."
They stay thin by "conscious consumption" —
an ongoing awareness of what they eat
and by the empowerment they gain
from that control.

"The Thinking Thin never go on a diet,
but they never go off one either."

This book reveals common sense tips and some of
the many simple adjustments to everyday eating and
lifestyle routines that this group consistently
practices to enjoy a lifetime of
weight control.

*National Center for Health Statistics at the Centers for Disease Control and Prevention. 2004.

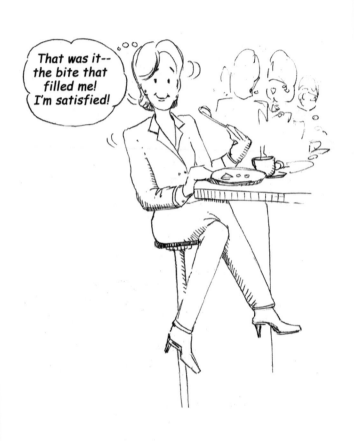

The Thinking Thin know
to listen to their bodies. They know there's
that one spoonful that will satisfy them —
after that, they're overeating.

❧

. . . *Hunger*

1.
The Thinking Thin believe
when they get hungry, it's an opportunity
to get their bodies working like efficient
fuel-burning machines.

2.
The Thinking Thin know hunger
is a sign that they need fuel. It's not
a feeling to deny or cause panic.

3.
The Thinking Thin know when the need
for fuel is met in the form of nutritious foods,
they will stop being hungry.

4.
The Thinking Thin
are calm about food.

5.

The Thinking Thin do not go to bed hungry.
They know a "little" nibbling before bed is OK.

6.

But The Thinking Thin know it's better to satiate
their hunger for a high carbohydrate during the day,
when their metabolism is in high gear, rather than later,
when their bodies slow down for the evening.

7.

The Thinking Thin do not "diet"
and do not deny themselves any food that they enjoy.
They do not put themselves in a "state of deprivation."
Instead, they watch their portions and monitor
their eating by the day.

8.

The Thinking Thin know it's easier to get
a read on their satiation if they eat s l o w l y.

9.

Many Thinking Thin believe when
they get hungry, their bodies hunt for fuel by
going into any "stored" food (better known as fat)
and "chew on that" for a while.

10.
The Thinking Thin know
sometimes, when they think they are hungry,
they are actually thirsty.

11.
The Thinking Thin practice
"conscious consumption."
(They are aware of everything they eat.)

12.
The Thinking Thin know
satisfaction is satiation, but not stuffed.
(They hate feeling stuffed!)

13.
When The Thinking Thin get hungry,
they consider all the healthy food options they
can choose, to fuel their bodies. Afterward, they feel
satiated and satisfied they've done something
nutritional for their bodies.

14.
The Thinking Thin know nature
provides a myriad of nutrients in fresh fruits
and vegetables and consuming lots of both
is a healthy way to stave off hunger.

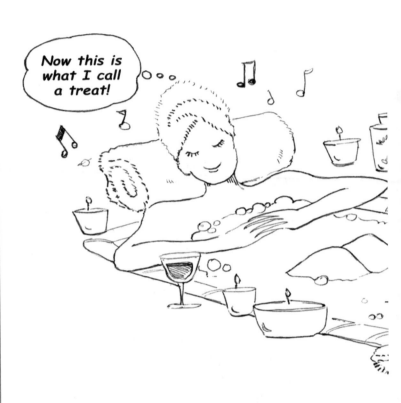

15.
*The Thinking Thin realize
what sets them apart from those
"who are not so happy with their weight"
is that they eat to "fuel their bodies"
and not "soothe their emotions."*

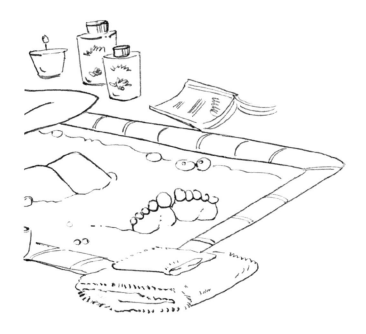

*Relaxing music, deep breathing,
a good soak, and a glass of wine (all at once)
are great for the emotions.*

16.
The Thinking Thin know hunger
is a body's signal that it needs nourishment.
They know they have to nourish, not just fill.
If they mindlessly eat, there is going to be a point
of satiation when their stomachs are filled
but their bodies are not
necessarily nourished.

17.
The Thinking Thin are guided
by their stomachs, but they do a little more
thinking about their food intake beforehand.
(Literally . . . before the hand puts
the food in the mouth!)

18.
Since The Thinking Thin eat lots
of nutritious foods, their desires for sweets
are often reduced and their hunger cravings are
usually not triggered by sugary foods.

19.
The Thinking Thin know hunger
is a chance to "use" foods as a way to keep
their bodies healthy. Food for fuel.

20.

*The Thinking Thin like to carry little mints
and pop them often. A minty mouth often deters
the addition of other foods for a while.*

21.

*The Thinking Thin do not avoid
their chocolate cravings. They enjoy chocolate
in small quantities.*

22.

*The Thinking Thin know that satisfying
hunger does not mean gorging on quantity.
They know they have to "fill up" or satiate
with the right kinds of food.*

23.

*Often, The Thinking Thin
will have a preplanned snack available
for when they know their hunger will kick in.
A banana ready at 11:00 a.m. is a good idea.*

24.

*The Thinking Thin find chewing gum
is a great way to cut cravings. It keeps the mouth
busy and the taste buds happy.*

Take one, please!

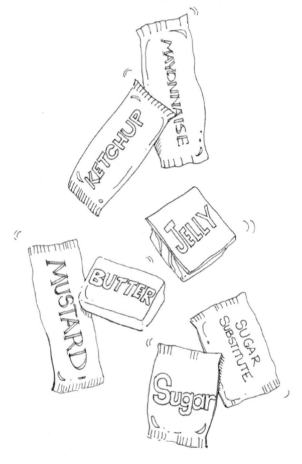

25.
*The Thinking Thin know it's important
how they manage the "freebies."*

❧

. . . *Portion Control*

26.
The Thinking Thin are thin because
they are not eating large quantities. Their bodies
can utilize what was just consumed and do not
have to store any extra consumption as fat.

27.
The Thinking Thin figure if they use
smaller plates, they will eat smaller portions.

28.
Most Thinking Thin can't even get the words
"Super-Size it, please" out of their mouths.

29.
The Thinking Thin like to take teeny bites
to help the flavor sensation last longer.
Even if it's a little bite-size candy. They refrain
from popping it in their mouths all at once.

30.
The Thinking Thin ask for lots of ice if a drink is
very sweet, knowing they will consume less sugar.

31.
The Thinking Thin could eat
the "large size" but they gratify their egos
(and hence their figures) before their stomachs.

32.
The Thinking Thin mentally "pre-portion" food
before they answer to their stomachs.

33.
Nosh \ `nawsch \ vb:` **to consume small quantities of a variety of foods**
The Thinking Thin know "nosh" is one of
the great words in their eating vocabulary and believe
it describes their eating routines, perfectly.

34.
The Thinking Thin enjoy immediate gratification,
if there is not too much of a long-term consequence.

35.
The Thinking Thin know one of the
best ways to curb consumption is to share a meal
with a friend. Portions are naturally halved
and this teaming makes for a great support duo.

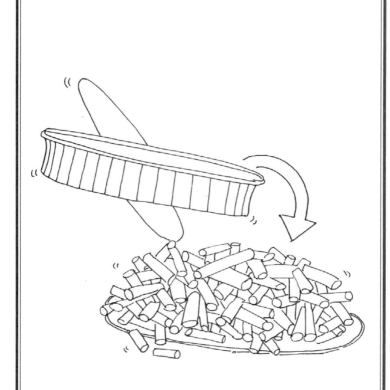

36.
The Thinking Thin notice that a lot of foods
that come in those round aluminum trays with
the corrugated sides probably contain quantities
beyond one serving size. They find it helpful to
transfer this food to a plate to see just
exactly how much they're getting!
*(Then they eat "one" portion
and save the rest.)*

37.

The

Thinking Thin

eat anything

they want;

they just

don't eat

all

of

anything!

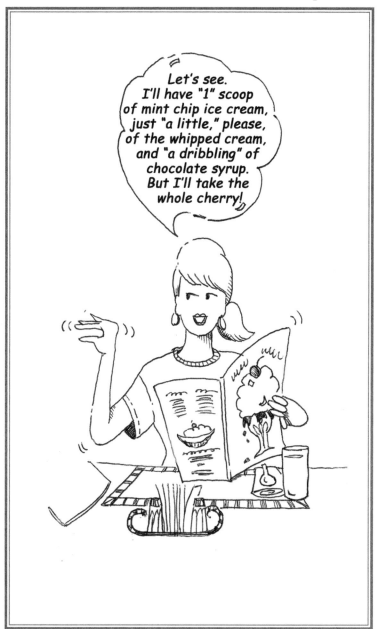

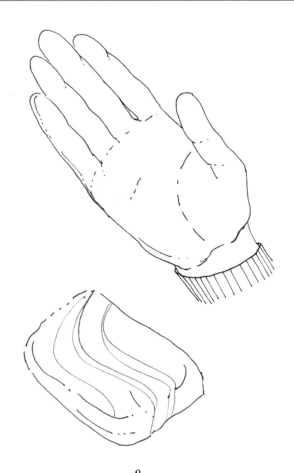

38.
*The Thinking Thin know a good rule
to keep at hand is to use the size of their palms
to determine a portion of food,
meat, for example.*

39.
The Thinking Thin control a high-fat
meal if it's put in front of them. They eat modest
portions of the high-fat food and consume more
of the low-fat component of their meal
— usually the side dish or salad.

40.
The Thinking Thin do not order large-size anything.
No large-size orders —> no large-size bodies!

41.
The Thinking Thin know to take "little" portions
of a lot of things so they aren't denying themselves.
Then they have a chance to taste everything —
"taste" being the operative word.

42.
The Thinking Thin know what Americans have
come to recognize as the size of an average meal is
TOO LARGE.

43.
The Thinking Thin get the "cup" of soup
and not the "bowl."

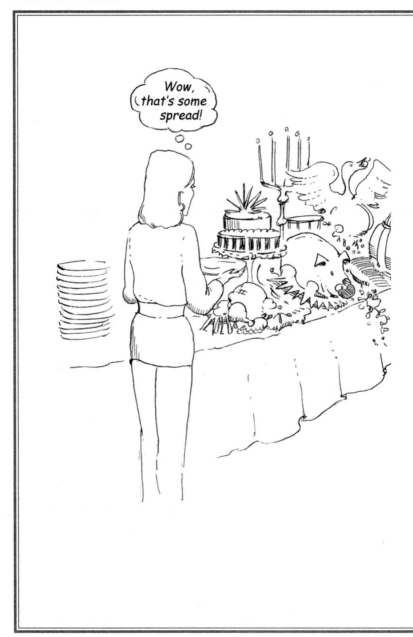

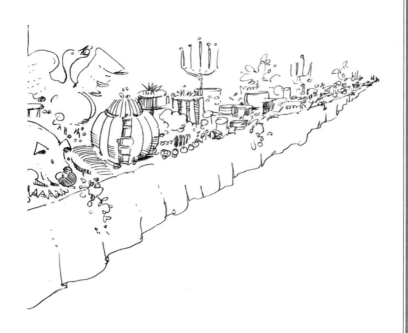

44.
*The Thinking Thin examine the food
at a buffet before they load their plates. Let's face it,
this is a "load the plate" situation, but they decide
beforehand what they want the most and mentally
"pre-portion" their serving sizes.*

45.
The Thinking Thin say

a "little" a lot.

46.
*The Thinking Thin get the smallest bag of chips
they can find to accompany their sandwich.*

47.
*The Thinking Thin know many restaurants
serve meals on 12" plates. Weren't they 9" plates
a few decades ago, when the American midsection
also had a smaller circumference?*

48.
*The Thinking Thin know it's a good idea
to store food in small portions. That way
they can eat the "whole thing" when in reality
they are eating a controlled portion.*

49.
*The Thinking Thin rarely use "substitute"
versions of food. They enjoy the real thing,
but they <u>watch the quantity</u>!*

50.
*The Thinking Thin believe airline portions
are just about the right amount of food. Yes they do.*

51.
*The Thinking Thin know the best way to empty
a box of chocolates is to serve it to guests, ASAP.*

Just about the right amount.

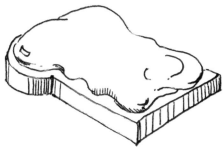

This is a bit overdone!

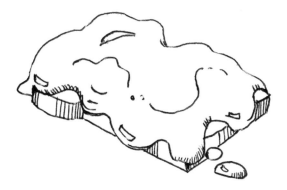

52.
*A lot of The Thinking Thin indulge in peanut
butter and jelly sandwiches, but they've learned
to spread both the pb and j sparingly.*

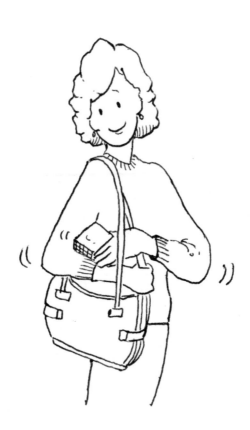

53.
*Often The Thinking Thin will save part
of their meal to eat at a later time in the day —
then they have something to look forward to.*

. . . Meals

54.
The Thinking Thin set food consumption goals
on a daily basis.

55.
The Thinking Thin think about food in the
framework of management. "I 'manage' my food."

56.
They know this daily management of their
food intake is the key to staying thin.
This is not a chore, it's a real confidence booster!

57.
The Thinking Thin think about what they are going
to eat before every meal, in terms of their hunger
and their nutrient needs. They like doing this;
it makes them feel in control.

58.
The Thinking Thin know how fattening
(and expensive) ordering out can be
if it's done frequently.

59.
The Thinking Thin believe that when those
"who are not so happy with their weight"
start to think and act like them, they will gradually
come to recognize high-fat, high-starch meals
as GROSS.

60.
The Thinking Thin know foods prepared in
a simple way are often the least fattening. (A squirt
of lemon is a great flavor enhancer to many foods.)

61.
The Thinking Thin do not panic when they overeat.
They sip water for a while — until that
full feeling subsides.

62.
The Thinking Thin know if they can still
see some of the design on their plate, it's a good
indication of a meal that's not too big.

63.
The Thinking Thin do not understand
"reduced-calorie" foods. They know "reduced-
calorie" wording could trick the mind into indulging.
They'd rather eat one serving of the real thing.

64.
The Thinking Thin know it's a major
bother to write down everything they eat
for a long period of time (even four days!).
They know it's better to have a consciousness about
what they're eating — by the day. Surely they remember
if they had a jelly-filled, sugar-coated doughnut at
breakfast to cut back on dessert at dinner.

65.
The Thinking Thin are prudent — by the forkful.

66.
The Thinking Thin do not look
at gaining weight as if it is a failure and figure
"What the heck, I've already ruined my diet —
I might as well have another." (Remember, The
Thinking Thin don't go on diets.) Extra weight is just
a little nuisance that they can take care of as soon
as they go back to their normal thinking.

67.
The Thinking Thin mentally barter foods all day —
questioning if they should consume certain foods,
based on what they previously ate.

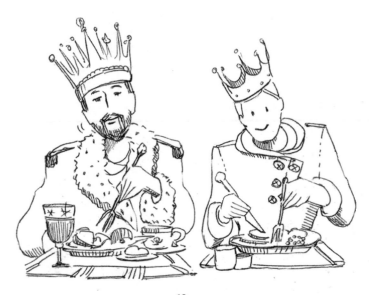

68.
The Thinking Thin know eating like
a "King for Breakfast, a Prince for Lunch . . .

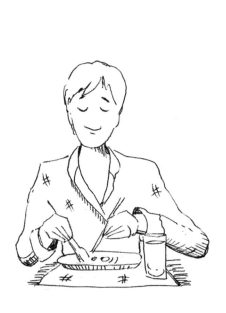

and a Pauper for Dinner" is a wise adage.

69.
Many Thinking Thin do not mind taking
a little extra time to prepare a nutritious meal
at home. They know exactly what they're eating and
the health benefits outweigh any inconveniences.

70.
The Thinking Thin try to eat dinner
at an early hour. This prevents them from filling up
on a heavy meal too late into the night and
going to bed with a full stomach.

71.
And they do not like to skip meals.
They know their bodies need consistent
sustenance for energy.

72.
The Thinking Thin are aware of the nutritional
value of the different components of their meal,
and they question whether together
they make up a balanced meal.

73.
The Thinking Thin are aware when
their drink and food have too much of the same
bad thing in them (salt or sugar, for example).
They curb their consumption of one or the other.

74.
The Thinking Thin know God did not build
the human body to survive predominately on
"meal substitutes." The Thinking Thin eat meals.

75.
The Thinking Thin know carrying
weight was nature's way of preserving fuel when,
as hunter/gatherers, we did not know where
our next meal was coming from — or when.
Most Americans pretty much know where
their next meal is coming from.

76.
The Thinking Thin often serve meals
on individual plates for each family member
and try to avoid serving dinners "family style,"
(serving dishes on the table). This way the temptation
to reach for second helpings is reduced.
This is time better spent talking and digesting.

77.
When confronted with a family-style meal,
The Thinking Thin make sure they
put just one serving on their plate.

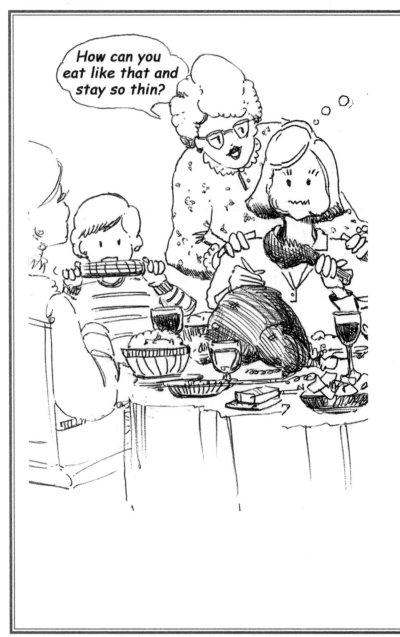

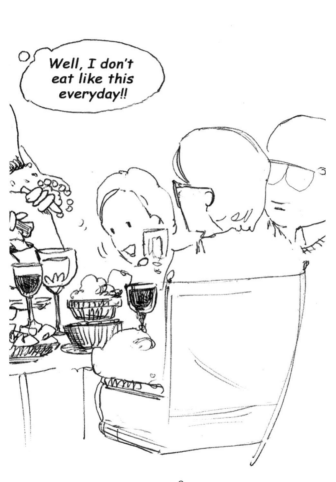

78.
*The Thinking Thin save indulging
for "special event" eating.*

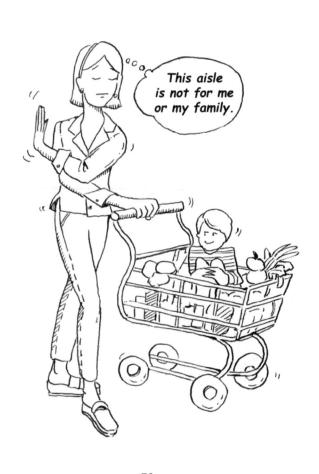

79.
The Thinking Thin are snobs about which foods they select for their families and themselves.

❧

. . . *Food Shopping*

80.
The Thinking Thin know they have a "choice"
when they select foods. This means they can pick
wisely from the many options on the grocery shelf.

81.
The Thinking Thin usually do not buy
a lot of prepared foods from the grocery store.
They are aware of all the additives —
especially hidden salts and sugars.

82.
The Thinking Thin know those "fruit" juice
drinks that make your tongue turn colors
are not so good for you. Many are mostly sugar.

83.
Many Thinking Thin often use
soy or soy products as a substitute for fattening or
high-cholesterol foods. They know this little bean
is a great source of protein.

84.
*The Thinking Thin explore foreign foods,
realizing there are many new and exciting sources
of vitamins and minerals. They know many exotic
countries developed local delicacies that
were nutritionally necessary for
their citizens' survival.*

85.
*The Thinking Thin know that there's
been a major increase not only in the amount
of packaged foods offered in the past 20 years,
but in the variety, and they can't help but notice
how this expansion of food types may have helped
expand the American girth.*

86.
*The Thinking Thin know monitoring the foods
they select from the grocery store is their family's
first defense against weight gain.*

87.
*The Thinking Thin food shop when they are
not hungry, then their selections are made from
a rational mind instead of a hungry stomach.*

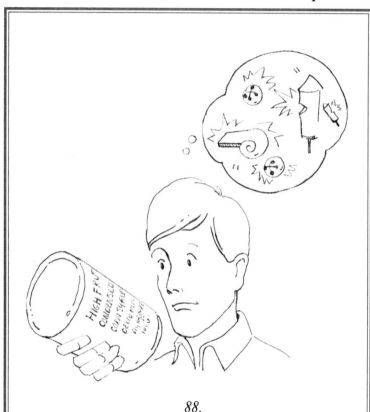

88.
The Thinking Thin read labels!
They know that the order of ingredients
is listed by the quantity. Seeing "sugar,"
"high-fructose," or "corn syrup" — and particularly
words they can't pronounce — near the top
of the list sets off alarms in their heads.

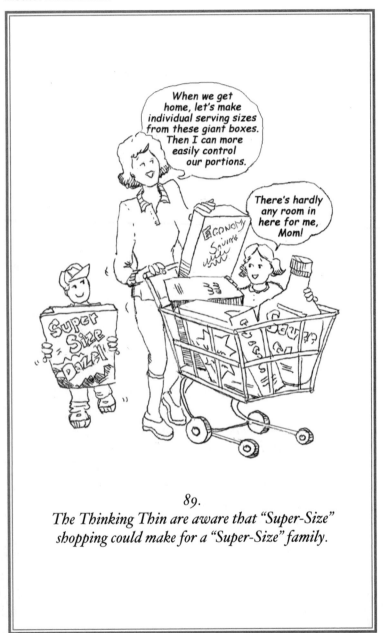

89.
The Thinking Thin are aware that "Super-Size"
shopping could make for a "Super-Size" family.

90.
Most Thinking Thin's grocery bags
have more fresh food purchases
than prepared foods.

91.
The Thinking Thin monitor their grocery lists.
They take notice if the items purchased
reflect a healthy diet — or not.

92.
A lot of Thinking Thin like
to make their basic food purchases first,
and then pick up any treats toward the end
of their shopping. This follows their normal
eating sequence, and allows them to better
monitor their treat allotments.

93.
The Thinking Thin like
to subdivide the large bulk-purchased
goods into smaller containers at home.
They store better in the kitchen and
prevent the temptation of large
portions because there is not
so much food visible.

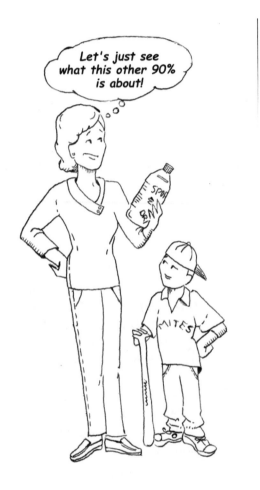

94.
*The Thinking Thin know that any drink that has
10% real fruit juice has 90% of something else!*

ॐ

. . . *Snacks*

95.
*The Thinking Thin know to manage their
intake of "treats" because the taste sensation
is short lived, and the consequence of indulging
sticks around — the waistline.*

96.
*The Thinking Thin try to eat only
one chocolate chip cookie (maybe two —
but only if they are small!). Their good self-image
is more gratifying than the indulgence.*

97.
*The Thinking Thin stop and think before
they select food. If they opt for an indulgent food,
they acknowledge this as an occasional "treat"
and enjoy it, guilt free.*

98.
*The Thinking Thin acknowledge their
cravings for snacks. To satisfy these, they look
for nutritious foods — often with protein —
like a little piece of cheese or chicken.*

99.
The Thinking Thin have a good habit for
(occasionally) eating crackers out of the box;
while they are still chewing (a small quantity),
their two hands are folding the wax paper
and closing the lid and putting
the box back in the cupboard.

100.
The Thinking Thin order "little gulps"
at convenience stores.

101.
The Thinking Thin learn certain food
combinations make a nice whole — part apple,
part cheese, part tomato, part avocado, for example.

102.
The Thinking Thin realize some chocolate-
covered ice cream bars that are twice the price
of others are also twice the portion! They often
choose to split these with a friend — because they
are too delicious to pass up.

103.
The Thinking Thin know nuts are nutritious
in small quantities.

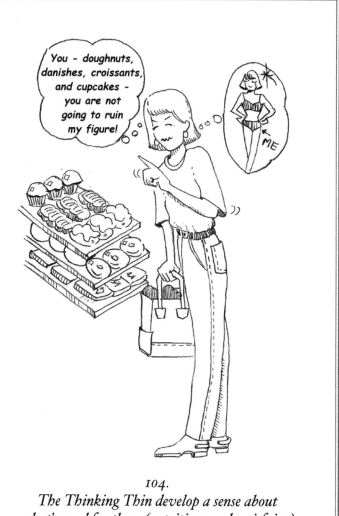

104.
*The Thinking Thin develop a sense about
what's good for them (nutritious and satisfying)
versus bad for them (just fillers to kill their hunger).
And if they're not sure, they eat half!*

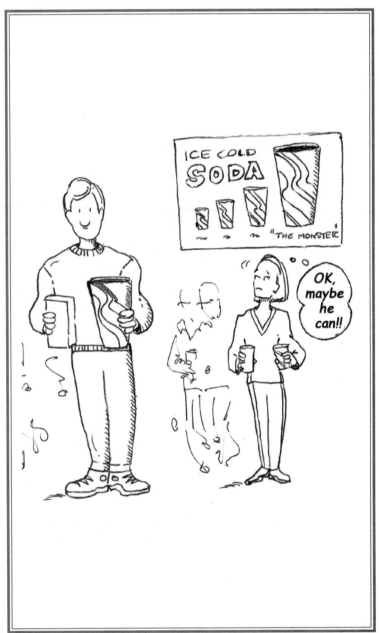

105.
The Thinking Thin don't know how anyone could finish that super-duper, gargantuan, mega-monstrous, megillah-size drink that the movie theaters offer.

106.
The Thinking Thin try not to buy
a lot of junk food during the day . . .

107.
instead, they like to have a "staple"
of nutritious treats they resort to. (An apple
and a little peanut butter is a good treat.)

108.
The Thinking Thin know when they get
the urge to splurge on chocolate rocky road ice
cream, they make sure they have a small dish ready
to serve it in — and not eat from the container.
(And using a small spoon helps to prolong
their eating enjoyment.)

109.
Sometimes The Thinking Thin
keep their eye on a "treat" but delay
consuming it until they can use it as a "reward."
They like to view little accomplishments,
even if it's a 15-minute walk,
as justification for a treat.

110.
The Thinking Thin learn to become
very sensitive to "sweet." They gradually decrease
their use of sugars and sweeteners. They learn
the more they use, the more they need to use.
So they learn to resort to the opposite --
the less they use, the less they need to use.

111.
The Thinking Thin know sugary sweets
are empty nutrition and that they'll
be hungry in a short while.

112.
The Thinking Thin are enticed by goodies,
just as much as everyone else: the chocolate cake,
the caramel ice cream, the sour cream,
the chive potato chips . . .

113.
but, they consider them a "treat" —
and consume them in small portions.

114.
The Thinking Thin know when they eat
an indulgent food, it is an occasional enjoyment
and not an eating staple.

115.

*The Thinking Thin know all
those snacks stacked up around the checkout
counter are positioned there for "impulse buying."
They turn a blind eye to these and stay focused
on their original intended purchase.*

116.

*Sometimes The Thinking Thin eat
vegetables like a piece of fruit. They can eat a pepper
or a tomato like an apple. OK, the seeds may drop
a bit and the tomato can get squishy, but they
just take a napkin — and a little packet of salt.*

117.

*The Thinking Thin love those
little bags of precut carrots, and they like
to keep them in a drawer at work.*

118.

*The Thinking Thin find cutting up fruits
and vegetables right after they get back from
the grocery store — and keeping them readily
available — curbs any temptation
to grab "bad" foods.*

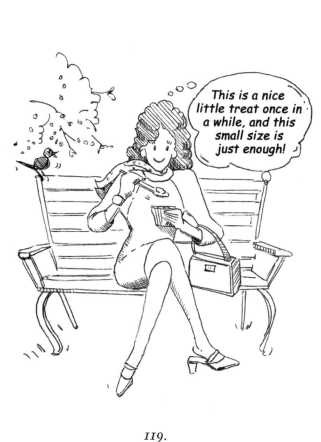

119.
The Thinking Thin do not try to justify soft frozen
desserts as diet helpers. Most are loaded with sugar.
(They put these in the treat category, and,
for goodness sake, they get the small!)

120.

*The Thinking Thin often treat their sweet tooth
to a snack that's sweet and healthy — raisins are
a great idea — and those little packs are so portable.*

121.

*The Thinking Thin enjoy a quick refresher —
a tall glass of ice water, a lemon slice,
and a "touch" of sweetener.*

122.

*And how easy are Popsicles made out of 100%
fruit juice? The Thinking Thin found a fun idea
is to stack a number of different flavors, by partially
filling the mold with one flavor, letting it freeze,
then repeating with different kinds (and colors)
of fruit juices. It's nutrition disguised
as a treat for kids.*

123.

*The Thinking Thin don't forget to count
condiments, too, in considering their daily intake.*

124.

*If The Thinking Thin do a little extra exercise
in their day, they allow themselves a little treat.*

125.
The Thinking Thin know snacks should
contain some protein and a little bit of carbs,
because these take longer to digest
and will stave off hunger.

126.
The Thinking Thin know there will always be
unhealthy food choices at arm's reach.
(They know they have control of
where their arms extend.)

127.
Often The Thinking Thin choose
the coffee-, lemon-, or vanilla-flavored yogurt
because it doesn't have all that sugary fruit at
the bottom that other flavor selections have.
And they know yogurt is an excellent
source of calcium.

128.
By saying "no" to sugary or salty snacks
more often than not, The Thinking Thin
know they are saying "yes" to a healthier
and more fit self.

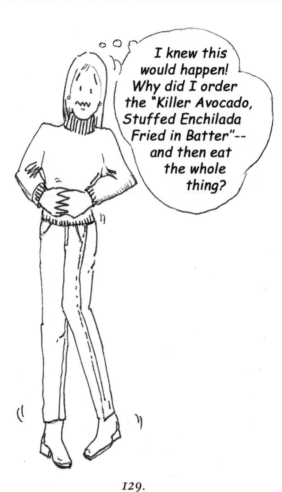

129.
The Thinking Thin are well aware
that most fast-food restaurants offer huge portions,
so there's a "sense" of value. They know if they eat
the whole thing there can often be a consequence.

❧

. . . Fast Foods

130.
Many of The Thinking Thin really do eat
at fast-food spots, because they know these restaurants
are now taking a stance on weight/health issues
and offer many healthy options.

131.
The Thinking Thin know these managed selections
and portions help them gain a sense of personal
empowerment for controlling their weight —
while still enjoying the foods they love.

132.
And they know fast foods are
a real treat for kids and a value for them.
They are aware that their children could emulate
their habits, so they are wise
with all selections.

133.
More likely than not,
The Thinking Thin get the small size —
then their bellies stay small!

134.
*The Thinking Thin often opt for foods
that are not fried or smothered in sauces.
And if they come that way, they know they can
always remove skins or push sauces aside.*

135.
*The Thinking Thin know a small-size soda at
fast-food restaurants looks suspiciously like the large-
size just a few decades ago. Hummmmmm.*

136.
*Most Thinking Thin love the burgers, the shakes,
and the french fries too! They just get the small size,
or have two of these three choices.*

137.
*The Thinking Thin know they occasionally
hunger for a **big, fat, juicy burger**. And have it!
(Then watch their consumption
for the rest of the day.)*

138.
*When in a fast-food restaurant, The Thinking Thin
know their "option to choose" is their most
powerful strategy for keeping themselves
in shape and maintaining good health.*

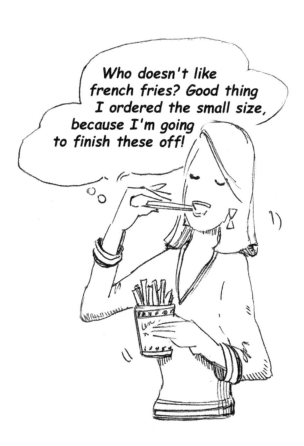

139.
The Thinking Thin eat all the french fries.
But they order the small size, because it's hard
not to polish them all off!

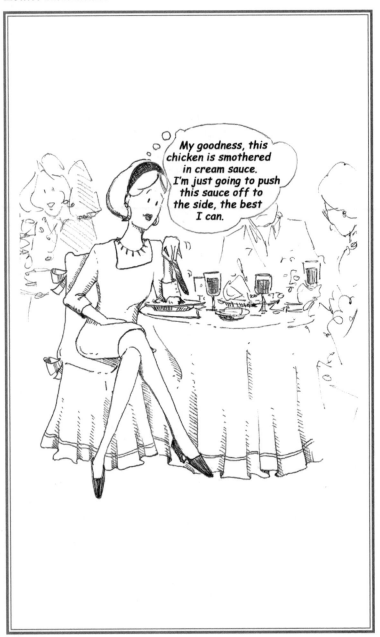

. . . Dining Out

140.
The Thinking Thin know the difference
between the "large-size" and the "small-size" order
is not deprivation. It's their smart choice.

141.
The Thinking Thin know they can't monitor
their food intake and then drink a lot of alcohol
and expect to manage their weight.

142.
The Thinking Thin do not
"get their money's worth" when they dine out.
They eat until they are satisfied
and don't stuff themselves.

143.
The Thinking Thin take a small amount of butter,
put it on their bread plate, and use only that.
They do not keep going back to the butter dish.
(Or they might lose track of how much
butter they're consuming.)

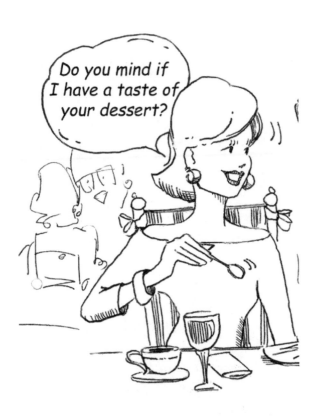

144.
*The Thinking Thin have a "taste"
of a dessert after a meal.*

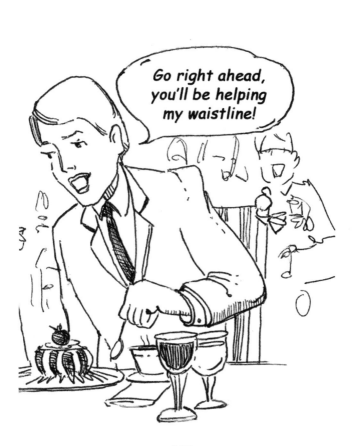

145.
Better yet, they prefer to "taste"
someone else's dessert after a meal.
(Because often just a spoonful
will do the trick!)

146.
*The Thinking Thin know
a "little" wine makes a meal enjoyable.*

147.
*When The Thinking Thin dine at a steakhouse,
they can pretty much expect the side dishes to be hearty
as well. They like to request the vegetable sides . . .
then attack the steak with gusto!*

148.
*The Thinking Thin evaluate their meals.
If their food has a lot of sugar in it, for example,
they will have a sugarless drink. If the meal has
two starches on the plate, they will be judicious
how much they consume of both.*

149.
*The Thinking Thin do not kid themselves by getting
a salad and then topping it with a rich dressing.*

150.
*The Thinking Thin try to order a vegetable,
salad, or light soup as an appetizer, knowing this
is an easier part of the meal in which to control the fat.
(Then they can enjoy a richer entrée if they want.)*

151.
The Thinking Thin sometimes have "spritzers"
because they know they're lessening their
consumption of alcohol proportionally
to the liquid they drink.

152.
When The Thinking Thin occasionally
enjoy fried food, they separate most of the skin from
the meat — and find it still tastes good.

153.
The Thinking Thin know a sweet potato
is a healthier option than a white potato. It's loaded
with good carbs and tons of fiber. And when zapped
in the microwave for six minutes, it's a quick and
delicious snack — just watch the toppings.

154.
The Thinking Thin know many popular chain
restaurants serve massive portions. Some pasta dishes —
that are considered one portion — can feed a family!
A rib dish might have a pound of meat
(almost five servings) and, with it, enough fries
for seven people! Oh my gosh!

155.
The Thinking Thin know eating out often
is the quickest way to pack on the pounds.

156.
Croutons absorb the dressing in a salad
and add unnecessary fat. The Thinking Thin skip
the croutons — or at least try to eat around them.

157.
The Thinking Thin believe
they are probably better off not using artificial
sweeteners. If they do, it's just a "little."

158.
Many of The Thinking Thin
prefer saltines or melba toast instead of
BREAD AND BUTTER
with their salad or meal.

159.
The Thinking Thin find that the best way
to limit their sugar consumption is to eat sweets
only after a meal. This way they are already
filled by the meal so they are satisfied with less.

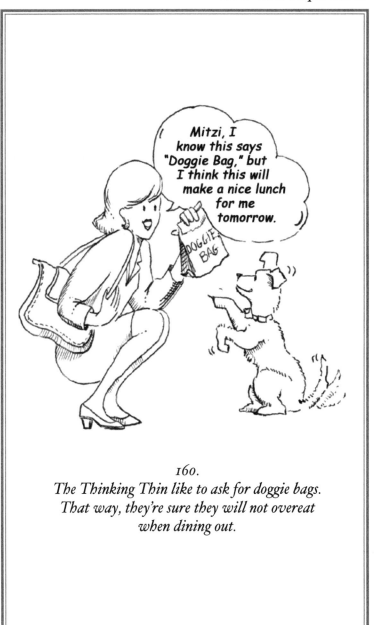

160.
The Thinking Thin like to ask for doggie bags.
That way, they're sure they will not overeat
when dining out.

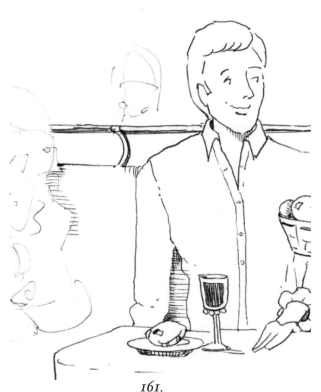

161.
The Thinking Thin know that filling up on bread
before a meal is a great dining-out casualty.
They usually find that one piece,
for the whole meal, is enough.

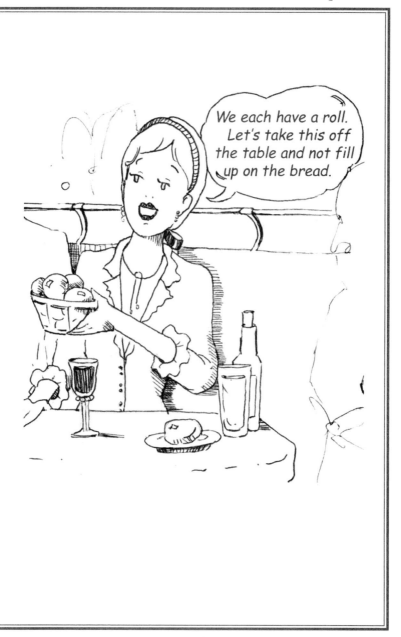

162.

The Thinking Thin avoid "All You Can Eat"
restaurants. This is the antithesis of their mind-set.
(But heck, once in a blue moon won't hurt.)

163.

The Thinking Thin know that at a dinner party
the food is prepared for their taste and enjoyment.
As guests, they allow themselves to enjoy —
then get back on track the next day.

164.

When dining out, The Thinking Thin
request a lot of orders "on the side."
They choose how much they want, not the chef.

165.

The Thinking Thin enjoy pasta occasionally,
but are careful with their sauce selections.
Red sauces with vegetables are excellent options.
Alfredo sauces, loaded with butter and cream,
might as well just jump
straight to the hips.

166.
When The Thinking Thin examine a menu,
they instinctively skip over the offerings
that contain offensive adjectives — "deep-fried"
being one of the scariest!

167.
The Thinking Thin may eat the sugary dessert —
or at least have a taste — but will not wash it down
with a sweet soda or very sweetened coffee.

168.
The Thinking Thin know restaurants
are in the business of making food taste great,
so the responsibility is up to individuals
to control their portions and intake of fat.

169.
The Thinking Thin find it's a good idea
to examine the entire menu, including the desserts,
when they order and to monitor their eating
as they fill up. If they are particularly looking
forward to the macadamia cheesecake,
they will go lightly on their appetizer
or entrée selection.

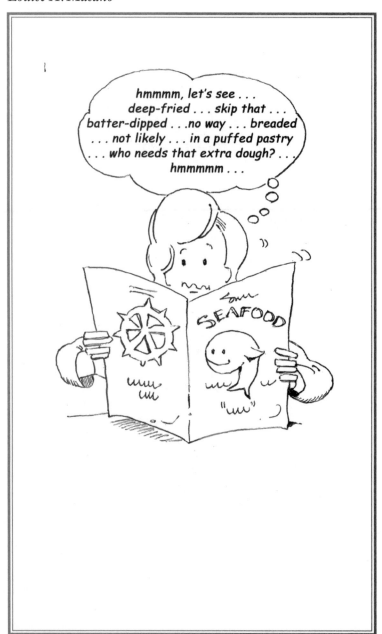

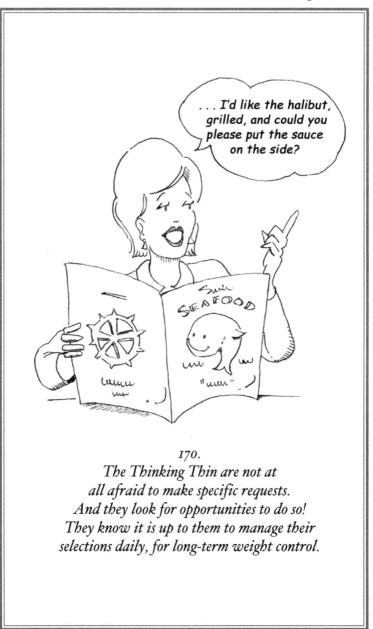

170.
The Thinking Thin are not at
all afraid to make specific requests.
And they look for opportunities to do so!
They know it is up to them to manage their
selections daily, for long-term weight control.

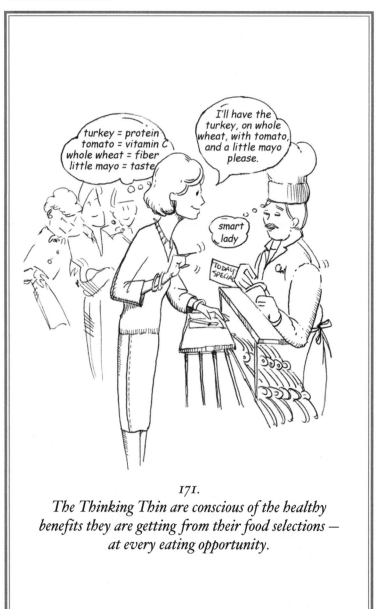

171.
The Thinking Thin are conscious of the healthy benefits they are getting from their food selections — at every eating opportunity.

❧

. . . *Breakfast & Lunch*

172.
The Thinking Thin know they have to eat
something in the morning to "fuel" their bodies.
This first eating of the day helps to kick in the body's
burning mechanism for the rest of the day.

173.
The Thinking Thin are selective
when they go to coffee bars. The rich coffee
specialties with all those enticing adjectives
are often loaded with sugar and fat!

174.
Because mornings are usually a rush,
The Thinking Thin know they have to pay
particular attention to the nutrition in their breakfast.
Coffee and sugary pastries give them
the dual impact of a caffeine and sugar buzz —
but it won't sustain them for very long.

175.
The Thinking Thin believe that
the breakfast plan shown on the back of some
cereal boxes is more than they eat in the morning.

176.

The Thinking Thin are leery of breakfast bars and snack bars. Many claim they are loaded with nutrients, but lots are also loaded with sugar — often added to mask the flavor of the vitamins and minerals.

177.

When The Thinking Thin have their first food of the day, they are aware of any special eating situation later in the day — like a birthday celebration — so they pace themselves.

178.

If some Thinking Thin treat themselves to cream and sugar in their coffee, they try to curb the amount of fat and sugar in the food that accompanies their coffee.

179.

Some clever Thinking Thin find it's a good idea to slice their bagels into thirds, instead of in halves. That way they're reducing their carbs and hardly noticing it! (And this thinner slice will not get stuck in the toaster.)

180.

The Thinking Thin add a lot of celery to their tuna salad to "bulk it up" without adding any fat.

181.
The Thinking Thin believe
that a muffin for breakfast is basically
a piece of cake! Cake for breakfast.
The Thinking Thin do not make a habit of this.
Occasionally, maybe, but they eat only half!
(And save the other half for later.)

182.
The Thinking Thin know cream of wheat and oatmeal
are great breakfast choices because of all that fiber.

183.
The Thinking Thin are aware that many "instant"
packets of oatmeal are often loaded with sugar!

184.
The Thinking Thin think it's an excellent habit
to drink a full glass of water first thing in the morning.
This is a good start to the eight glasses
they like to have throughout the day.

185.
The Thinking Thin drink their eight glasses of water
as follows: first thing in the morning, mid-morning,
before lunch, early afternoon, late afternoon,
before dinner, mid-evening,
and right before bed.

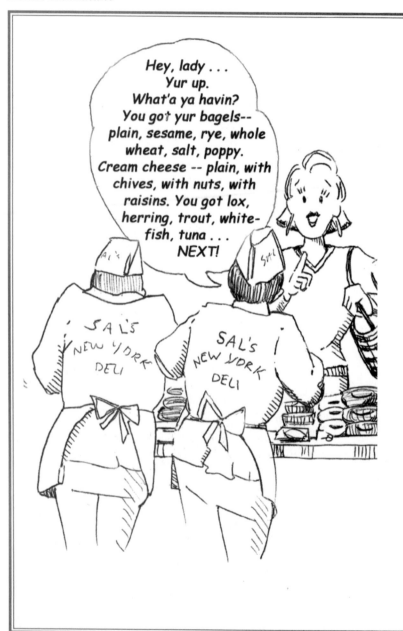

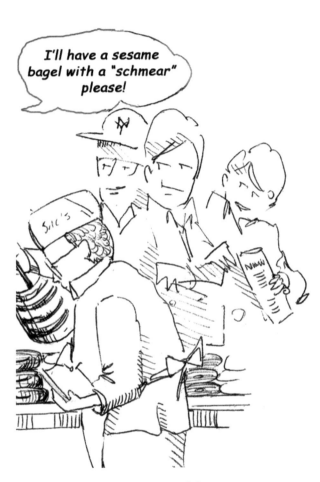

186.
Some Thinking Thin in New York City
order their bagels with a "schmear."
(Translation: cream cheese spread quickly
and lightly over a bagel.) Then they eat half.

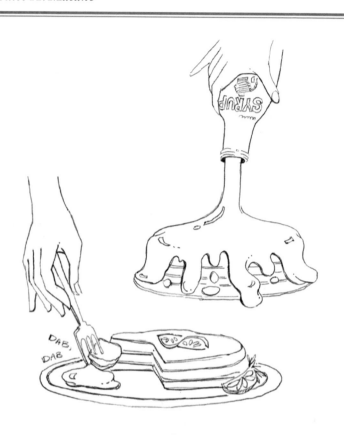

187.
*The Thinking Thin know pancakes are
a special treat. They often opt for the buckwheat
kind because they are loaded with good carbs.
And they watch out about <u>drenching</u> them
in maple syrup! They find it best if they pour
a bit of syrup on their plate and judiciously
dab a forkful of pancake at a time.*

188.
A one-minute breakfast: An egg in a cup
(out of the shell, please!), zapped in the microwave
for 35 seconds, is cooked without fat or butter.
(And could probably be eaten in under that time!)

189.
The Thinking Thin know hot dogs taste
extra great at a ball game. This is "event" eating
and they have no qualms about enjoying them
with "everything."

190.
About the fruit at the bottom of that low-fat yogurt —
doesn't that look an awful lot like two tablespoons
of jelly? The Thinking Thin mix it in sparingly,
and do not scrape it all up from the bottom!

191.
The Thinking Thin know eggs are loaded
with protein and are a nutritious breakfast,
but they often eat more "whites" than "yokes."

192.
The Thinking Thin choose gyms close to their work.
Then they have three opportunities a day to go for
a workout — before work, after work, or lunchtime.

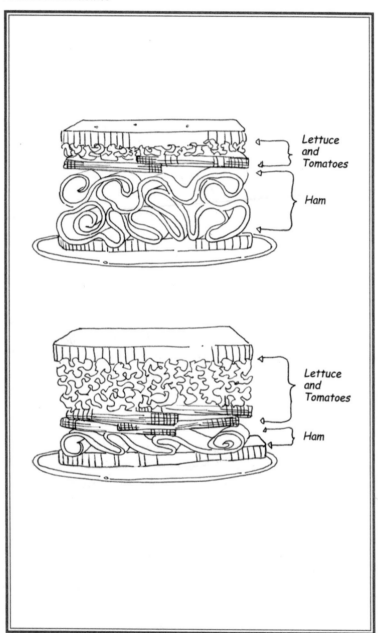

193.

The

Thinking Thin

proportion

their sandwiches

to favor

the healthier

components.

194.
The Thinking Thin enjoy an occasional slice
of pizza and often choose the vegetable toppings
over the meat options. Then they feel they make
a treat into a healthy choice.

195.
The Thinking Thin know that chef salads
aren't necessarily healthy because they can be
loaded with hidden fats — all that meat and cheese!
And they watch the fattening dressings!
(A little oil and vinegar are a safe choice.)

196.
The Thinking Thin spend some time
at the deli counter, looking for nutritional options.
They select bird meats (turkey and chicken)
before animal meats (cows and pigs).
Also grain breads are better than white.
And they watch that mayo.

197.
The California Burger originated from
a West Coast health consciousness.
The Thinking Thin opt for this selection
often because it can replace a cheese
or bacon topping with tomato and lettuce.

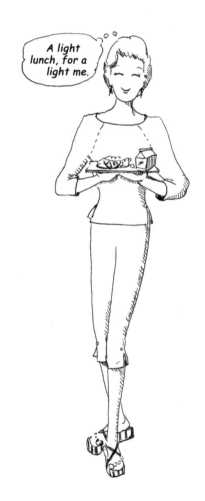

198.
The Thinking Thin's figures match
the amount of food they take in.

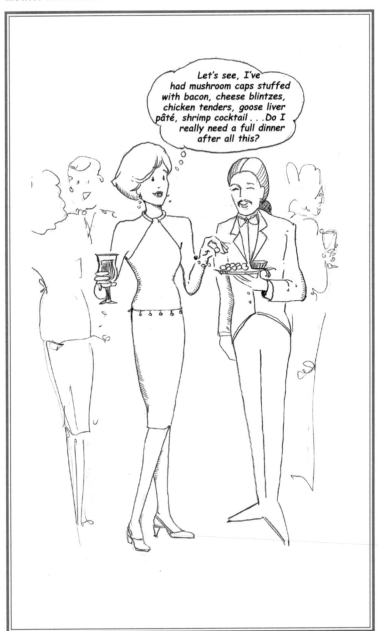

❧

. . . *Parties*

199.
The Thinking Thin reach
for the smallest hors d'oeuvre.

200.
The Thinking Thin count cocktail food
as part of their evening's food intake. (Yes, it counts —
even if they're standing up and nibbling.)

201.
The Thinking Thin know parties
are an easy route to "mindless munching"
and they are on extra high alert
in monitoring their intake.

202.
The Thinking Thin keep in mind that hors
d'oeuvres are presented BEFORE a meal,
when they are naturally very hungry
and their stomachs are empty.
They consciously limit these, knowing
there is a meal soon to follow.

203.
Also, a meal with hors d'oeuvres is probably special and served a little later than the norm, making for extra hungry guests!

204.
Hummus is flavored chickpeas — loaded with fiber — an excellent dip.

205.
Often when The Thinking Thin order a drink, they also order a glass of ice water and drink both intermittently. This controls the intake of alcohol and cuts down on inebriation.

206.
Many young Thinking Thin realize most parties serve only alcoholic drinks and salty snacks. They like to eat a well-balanced meal beforehand, to prevent the consumption of too much party food and drink.

207.
The Thinking Thin nibble on any fruits or vegetables offered first, before they dive into those mini hot dog appetizers.

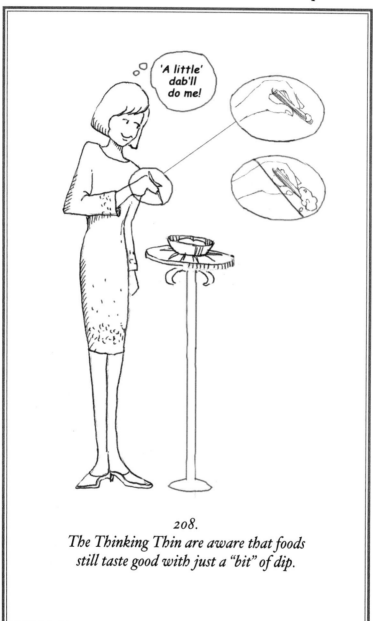

208.
The Thinking Thin are aware that foods still taste good with just a "bit" of dip.

209.

*When The Thinking
Thin order a mixed
drink, they ask for
more "mix"
than
drink.
"Light
on the
liquor,
please!"*

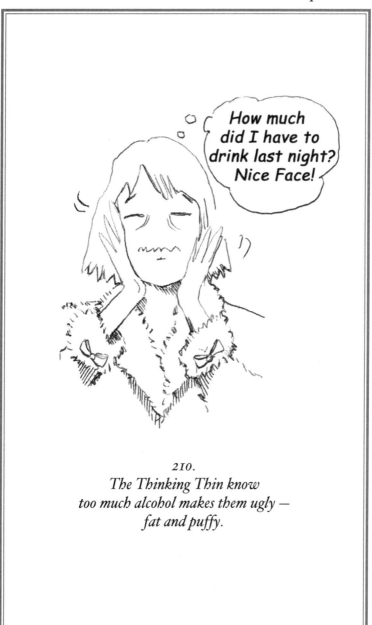

210.
The Thinking Thin know
too much alcohol makes them ugly —
fat and puffy.

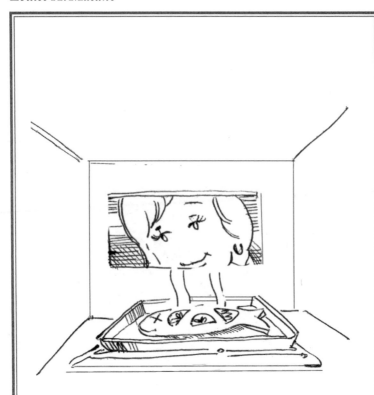

211.
*The Thinking Thin know the oil from fresh fish,
particularly salmon, is excellent for them.
(And it's healthier to broil or bake than fry!)*

. . . *Food at Home*

212.
*The Thinking Thin like to redo their cupboards
and rid themselves of huge plates, bowls, and glasses —
or at least shove them to the back of the shelf.
Large plates encourage large portions.*

213.
*The Thinking Thin know that if
the condensed soup calls for one can of milk,
they can use a half can of milk and a half can
of water and hardly notice the difference.
They cut back on the fat from the milk
and the consistency is still pretty true
to the soup company's intent.*

214.
*The Thinking Thin know apple pieces
make a delicious "sweetener" to a vegetable mix.
Nature pretty much figured out how
to keep our taste buds happy.*

215.
The Thinking Thin slice meats "thin."

216.
The Thinking Thin learn to use fresh herbs
to enhance food instead of a lot of butters, salts,
fattening dressings, and rich sauces.

217.
The Thinking Thin find they can enhance
an eating experience by appealing to all five senses.
They get out the pretty plates, play some
soothing music, fill their home with delicious smells,
embellish the food with fabulous seasonings,
and even consider food that needs
one's hands to "touch."

218.
The Thinking Thin like to keep a full bottle
of water in the refrigerator — in the same spot.
In the door shelf is a good idea. (Then they can
blindly grab the bottle and take frequent swigs.)

219.
The Thinking Thin will often cut up leftovers
to store in many one-serving-size portions.
This way, when they raid the fridge,
they are grabbing only one
pre-measured portion.

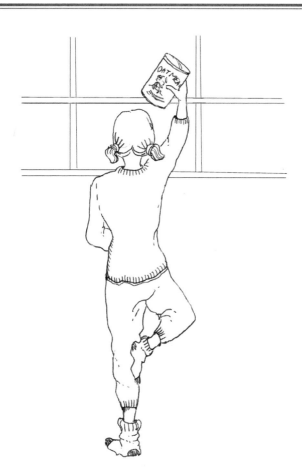

220.
The Thinking Thin like to always have
a few nutritious, non-perishable foods handy
for when their cupboards are nearing bare.
Oatmeal, the kind in the round canister,
is a good choice.

221.
The Thinking Thin like to skin
their chicken breasts (or buy them like that).
Most of the fat is right under the skin.

222.
When they cook, The Thinking Thin like
to munch on raw vegetables (dipped in a bit
of olive oil and pepper). This is particularly good
when baking sweets. The two different tastes
help prevent dipping into the sweet batter.

223.
The Thinking Thin find it's a good idea to measure
oils and shortening accurately to control portions.
Randomly pouring or slicing can add
unnecessary extra fat.

224.
The Thinking Thin have learned
that "bad carbs" are often identified as "white foods"
that are easy to chew, for example, white bread,
instant white rice, and white potatoes.

225.
The Thinking Thin think grilling is great,
because it eliminates the need for cooking
in unnecessary oils. (They also make friends
with the broiler and learn to poach.)

226.
The Thinking Thin keep their eyes out for
recipes that have clever ways to create flavorful,
healthy meals with interesting food combinations.

227.
The Thinking Thin like to "juice," then they
are confident of the pure ingredients in their drinks.

228.
A lot of The Thinking Thin are capable
of preparing three or four quick, nutritious meals.
Then they don't have to resort to eating out
or ordering in so often.

229.
Sometimes The Thinking Thin
can't even find the sugar in their cupboards.

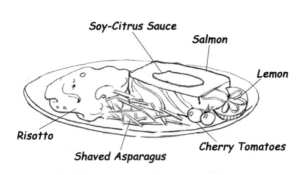

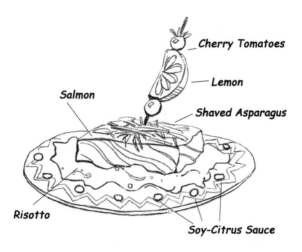

230.
The Thinking Thin know how appealing
an average meal can be when it is stacked high.
This is a simple, artful technique they can do at home.
(Just like a fancy restaurant would serve it.)

231.
The Thinking Thin find chilled
cottage cheese with some fresh fruit cut up
and mixed in (served in one scoop!) can compete
with almost any sugary dessert.

232.
The Thinking Thin know bread made
from unbleached, enriched wheat flour is healthier
than bleached white flour. Certain breads
offer good opportunities to add
nutrients to a meal.

233.
The Thinking Thin prefer to use
fats that are liquid at room temperature
(vegetable oils, for example) over fats that are solid
at room temperature (like butter and lard).

234.
The Thinking Thin know when
their refrigerators are stocked with fresh fruits
and vegetables they are better able
to maintain a healthy lifestyle for
their families and themselves.

235.
The Thinking Thin find it's a good idea
not to transport whole boxes, cans, or cartons
of food with them from the kitchen to the TV room.
They make a serving on a platter and transport that.
This preset portion curbs overeating.

236.
The Thinking Thin know TV programs
and commercials greatly influence eating behavior.

237.
The Thinking Thin know more money
is spent on advertisements for fast food than on
advertisements for fresh fruits and vegetables.

238.
The Thinking Thin realize they do not need
most of the food products that are out there.

239.
The Thinking Thin disregard most advertising
claims that brag about quick weight loss.

240.
Just because there are a lot
of happy people in commercials for restaurants
does not necessarily mean they consume all these foods.
Most actors watch what they eat —
to stay telegenic.

241.
The Thinking Thin try to stay
mindful of how recently they had their last meal
when they decide to eat in front of the TV.
Sometimes a small snack is all they need.

242.
When The Thinking Thin are in
a gorging mood, they microwave popcorn
and munch to their heart's delight.
And they watch the butter!

243.
The Thinking Thin know
a pizza in front of the TV
is a meal, not a snack.

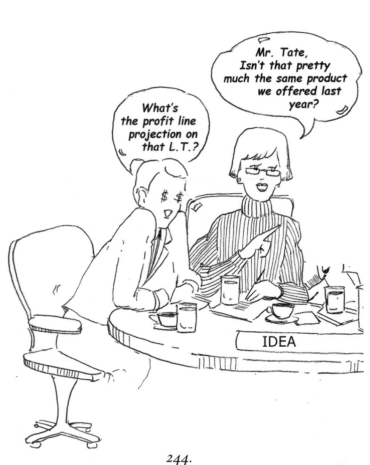

244.
The Thinking Thin know a lot of companies that pitch "quick weight loss" products are mostly thinking about the profits they are going to make.

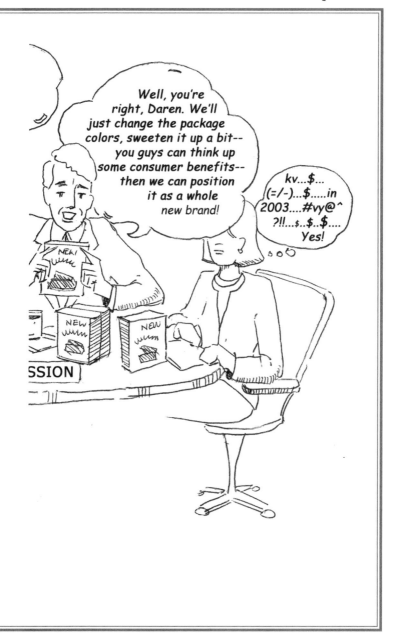

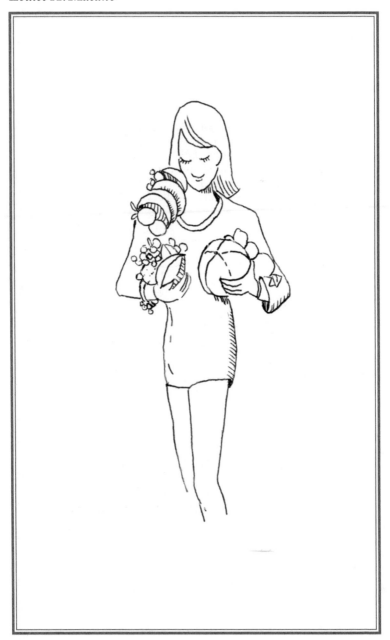

. . . *Food Choices*

245.
*The Thinking Thin anticipate the flavor
and nutrient value of foods they "choose."*

246.
*The Thinking Thin know
they have a choice of what they select to eat.
And realize that people who say they are too busy
with their jobs and their kids to eat right
are still making choices . . .
to eat wrong!*

247.
*The Thinking Thin know
that people are busier than ever before.
(Probably because more women are in the
workforce and they often have to do double time
with the housework and kids.) This should not
be an excuse for bad food choices.
It is just a lack of awareness
of what one is consuming.*

248.
*The Thinking Thin know it's just as
easy to pick up an apple as it is a candy bar.
It's usually cheaper and just as portable.
And they enjoy the apple's nutritional value
over the candy bar's sweetness. They feel good
about doing something healthy for their bodies,
knowing they are getting both taste <u>and</u> nutrition.*

249.
*The Thinking Thin know condiments count
and, if given the choice, will select mustard
over ketchup or mayonnaise. (Most ketchups
are loaded with sugar and mayo is high in fat.)*

250.
*The Thinking Thin are very much
aware of the dangers of drinking alcohol,
and not just because of how fattening it is.
They realize that inebriation lets down their defenses,
including their sound judgment about the amount
of food they are consuming while they drink.
Staying sober helps
keep them thin.*

251.
When The Thinking Thin use cream in
their coffee — it's a modest amount. (Sometimes they
use part cream and part whole or skim milk.)

252.
The Thinking Thin know the United States
has one of the best agricultural, food manufacturing
and food distribution systems in the world
and they can get just about anything, anytime,
and anyplace they want. They realize what lucky folks
they are to live in such an abundant place and time,
and know these choices are theirs not to abuse.

253.
The Thinking Thin and fish are one!
They know fish is good food and feel good eating
lots of it. They eat fish to live longer.

254.
Fish is a diet staple in many countries that
don't seem to share this country's weight problem.
The Thinking Thin try to eat fish
three to four times a week.

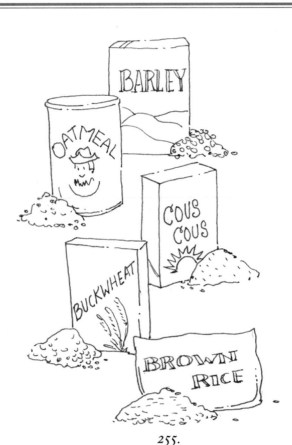

255.
The Thinking Thin know there are
good carbs and work these into their daily intake.
Good carbs give the body a slow-burn energy.
(As opposed to bad carbs, which shoot up
the blood sugar and then drop it like a rock.)
Good carbs are unrefined grains, brown rice,
oatmeal, barley, couscous, risotto, and buckwheat.
And these are packed with vitamins and minerals
which can help to stave off hunger.

256.
The Thinking Thin wonder,
"Did anyone ever lose weight on low-fat cookies?"
They prefer to buy regular cookies and eat one or two.
The low-fat kinds encourage indulgence.

257.
And they don't keep cookies on shelves
that are at eye level. This high visibility creates
unnecessary temptation.

258.
The Thinking Thin know to eat moderate
portions of foods that formerly had four legs.

259.
The Thinking Thin know kids like sweets.
Kids have kids' tastes. The Thinking Thin know
they don't have to eat their kids' food.

260.
The Thinking Thin try to have at least
three to four servings of fruits or vegetables a day.
They look for new varieties that add diversity
to their meals and snacks.

261.

The Thinking Thin know butter
is fattening and high in cholesterol. But it tastes
so much better than those frightening substitutes.
Oh heck, they like to use the real thing
— but not too much!

262.

The Thinking Thin know broiled IN the oven
is better than fried ON the stove top.

263.

The Thinking Thin know fried
is a four-letter word with an extra letter.

264.

The Thinking Thin believe foods that
grew in the ground are probably a better choice
than foods that walked on the ground.

265.

The Thinking Thin are very careful
about the liquids they put into their bodies.
A lot of popular juices and soft drinks
contain a tremendous amount of sugar.

266.
The Thinking Thin know the standard
food pyramid they learned in grade school is still
a good basis for daily consumption. Lots of fruits
and vegetables, whole grains and legumes, and
smaller portions of animal foods (meat and dairy).

267.
The Thinking Thin know they can fill up on
nutritious foods as easily as they can on fatty foods.

268.
Before The Thinking Thin open
their refrigerator doors, they like to have
a plate handy to hold their "portioned" selections.
This discourages eating right from the containers.

269.
The Thinking Thin know some popular vegetable
juices contain almost a full day's recommendation
of salt intake in just one serving. Wow, that's a lot!

270.
Many of The Thinking Thin's favorite food color
is green — all those delicious garden vegetables
loaded with vitamins and minerals.

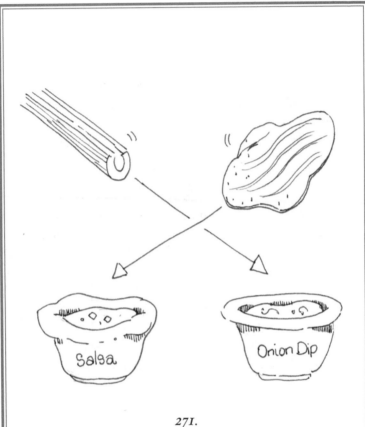

271.
Some Thinking Thin control hors d'oeuvres by
"cross-referencing." As an example, celery has no fat,
so they can treat themselves to a "bit" of a high-fat dip.
And conversely, if they "need that chip,"
they will opt for the salsa, or a lower-fat dip.
(The best of both worlds is to use
the celery with the salsa.)

272.
The Thinking Thin know a lot of prepared
and canned foods are REALLY SALTY,
even if they can't taste it.

273.
The Thinking Thin indulge their taste buds
with flavor, not their stomachs with volume.

274.
The Thinking Thin prefer honey over sugar
in their tea. It makes them feel healthy.

275.
The Thinking Thin get excited by fruits.
They're great at room temperature, but cold
from the fridge can compete with most desserts.
Cold, fresh melons, berries, peaches,
apricots, etc. — delicious!

276.
The Thinking Thin believe that extra slice
of bread in a club sandwich is totally unnecessary.
(And bet they wouldn't miss it if it wasn't there.)

277.

The Thinking Thin eat the bacon.
They eat one or two pieces, and they nibble
around the fat -- it is possible because they can
see the line between the meat and the fat.
They're still getting that good smoky taste —
and they didn't eat the fat.

278.

The Thinking Thin know flavored seltzer
water is a great alternative to a sweetened soda.
It's still carbonated, but it's sodium-free,
sugar-free, and so refreshing.

279.

The Thinking Thin often carry a little piece
of (wrapped!) candy in their purses or pockets.
This is a nice treat to have "at the ready"
and often reduces the urge to stop
and buy a more indulgent treat.

280.

The Thinking Thin know the proliferation
of "low-fat" and "diet" products is not reflected
in the national waistline. They realize <u>only they</u>
have the power to decide how they want to look!

281.
The Thinking Thin take time
at the store to look for drinks without sweeteners.
They know the sweeteners in non-diet soft drinks
are a major source of unnecessary sugar,
do not satiate hunger, and might make
them hyper. Really bad.

282.
The Thinking Thin know that gas station
convenience stores have one of the worst ratios
of healthy food to junk food. They're terrible!
But with a little creative thinking,
they can actually find some healthy choices.
They look for bottled water, unsweetened
fruit juices, or seltzers, protein snacks
like nuts, yogurt, or a bit of cheese.
(If the food choices are really dismal,
they opt for the less offensive pretzels.)

283.
The Thinking Thin know the portable foods
that come in nature's convenient wrappers . . .
bananas, nuts, oranges, mangos, etc.
are usually very nutritious.

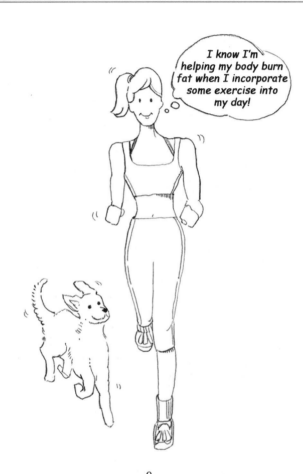

284.
The Thinking Thin don't credit
their metabolism for their weight success.
They often "speed up" the fat-burning process
with some physical activity.

. . . *Being Active*

285.

*The Thinking Thin like to start each day
with a lively step — even if they are just walking
to their car. They are conscious
that their body is burning fuel.*

286.

*The Thinking Thin know everyone
cannot be a super athlete. And that all those
high achievers they read about in magazines
are the exception, not the rule (but good for them!).
A ten-minute walk incorporated into their day,
where there was not one before,
is a great achievement.*

287.

*The Thinking Thin know they have
to make time to be physically active.
Even if it seems like a chore, they try
to recall beforehand how good
they feel after they are active.
This helps them get going.*

288.
The Thinking Thin know sometimes
when people say, "I don't have time," they should
just check how much time, for instance, they spend
on the phone. Perhaps there are ten minutes right there
that would be better spent walking around the block.
Good time to put a cell phone to optimal use —
talk and walk. (Watch the traffic, though!)

289.
The Thinking Thin know
exercise alone won't make them thin.
They watch their consumption.

290.
The Thinking Thin know that domestic animals
can get fat because they are not outside roaming.
They are creatures of interiors — kind of like
Americans with TV and video gizmos.

291.
The Thinking Thin know an increase
in physical activity will increase their appetite
and a few healthy snacks throughout the day
will boost their energy and hold off
their hunger until mealtime.

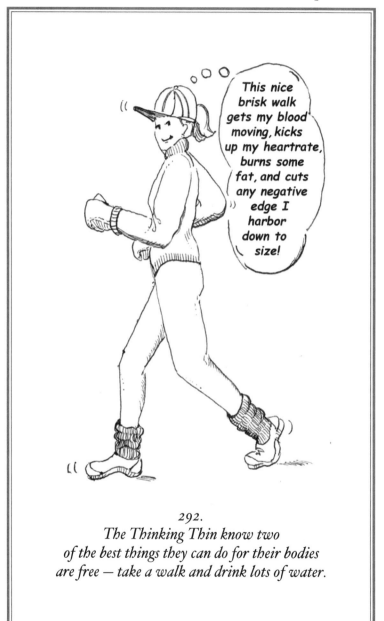

292.
The Thinking Thin know two
of the best things they can do for their bodies
are free — take a walk and drink lots of water.

293.
The Thinking Thin barter exercise for food.
If they decide to indulge in a treat, they know
to add a little extra physical activity to their day.
A walk around the block, a quick sprint up
the stairs, a few minutes running in place . . .

294.
The Thinking Thin find a daily five-
or even three-minute jog in place is easily doable
and helps make them feel energetic.

295.
The Thinking Thin know the body
tries like heck to get itself healthy.

296.
The Thinking Thin make sure they get
the appropriate amount of exercise to balance
occasional (allowable) "big eating."

297.
The Thinking Thin know it's possible
to balance food intake and exercise activities
and are conscious of their daily
utilization of both.

298.
The Thinking Thin realize their body is like an
efficient fuel-burning car. They give it what it needs.
A car was designed to efficiently utilize fuel from
the gas tank — and not to carry it somewhere else
on the car for later use. Carrying extra gasoline
can be dangerous! Like carrying extra fat!

299.
The Thinking Thin notice how happy pets
are to get out and run about and they have
this same appreciation for being active.

300.
The Thinking Thin are not bummed out
if there is not a parking space right out front.
They are just as happy to park far away and look
forward to the walk for a bit of unexpected exercise.

301.
The Thinking Thin like to go
and get their own lunch. They look at this
as an opportunity to get some exercise,
knowing they are burning "fuel" before
they take in more food.

302.
The Thinking Thin do not like
to pass up an opportunity to get out
in the fresh air and do activities.

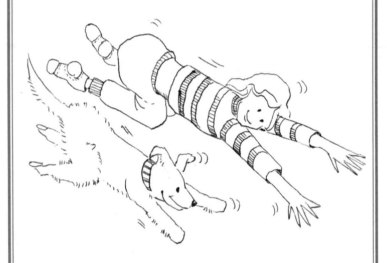

303.
The Thinking Thin know
they can learn from the animals.
Many animals stretch when they wake up.
Nature did all the thinking for them,
and we're left to our own devices!

304.
The Thinking Thin are not slaves to the gym.
They go because it makes them feel good,
not because they will gain massive amounts of weight
if they don't go. They try to get little bits of exercise
in a lot of different ways throughout their day.

305.
Many Thinking Thin know a TV
commercial break is a good time to stand up
and stretch, rather than run to the refrigerator.

306.
The Thinking Thin know 10 to 20 sit-ups a day
at home can contribute to a tighter stomach.

307.
The Thinking Thin like to silently do isometrics
at their desks at work. What a great way
to exercise without getting up.

308.
The Thinking Thin know lifting weights,
even a modest amount (five to ten pounds)
a few times a week, is wonderful for
their metabolism and bone density.

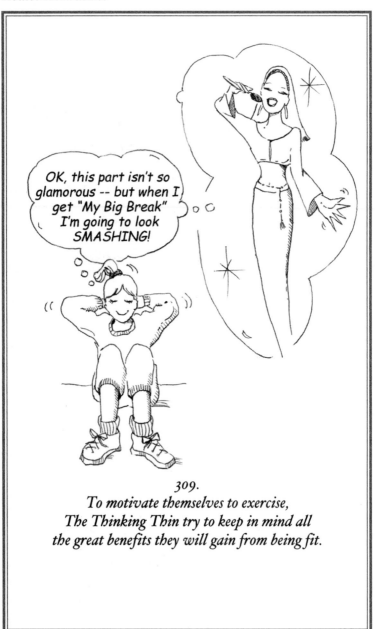

309.
To motivate themselves to exercise,
The Thinking Thin try to keep in mind all
the great benefits they will gain from being fit.

310.
The Thinking Thin know you don't have
to be thin to run a marathon, but "fit" is a must.

311.
The Thinking Thin know a fit body is a by-product
of healthy eating and an active lifestyle.

312.
The Thinking Thin take the stairs with gusto.
They like to think of the word "bound."

313.
The Thinking Thin know body types
(bone and muscle configurations) vary.
But a healthy, toned body is a winner
above all else.

314.
The Thinking Thin find yoga is
a wonderful discipline to learn — with effective
results that contribute to their overall mental
and physical well-being.

315.
*The Thinking Thin like to add
a little "pep to their step."*

316.
*Some of The Thinking Thin like to do stretches
whenever they can — extending legs under the desk,
flexing ankles and releasing, raising arms above
their heads to elongate their back muscles,
taking a few minutes to stand and touch the floor
with their fingertips and if they can, palms.*

317.
*The Thinking Thin know muscle weighs
more that fat. So if they are more physically
active, thus gaining muscle and losing fat,
they may not necessarily see much
weight difference on the scale.*

318.
*The Thinking Thin know if they are
physically active — even just 20 minutes a day —
they are adding tremendously to a healthy
and possibly longer life.*

319.
The Thinking Thin would rather walk than ride.
This is a nice way to pick up some good vitamin D
from the sun, for that "sun-kissed" look.
(A light sunscreen is a must.)

320.
The Thinking Thin like to swing their hips
when they walk because they get a little extra
waist twist. Plus the longer strides get them
to their destination more quickly!

321.
The Thinking Thin know being aerobic
and getting the blood moving gives them
(and anyone) one of their best looks
— a natural glow.

322.
The Thinking Thin know those slant boards
at gyms are wonderful. They lie inclined
with their head at the lower end, then
their blood can circulate to their complexion.
They look at this relaxation as a treat after
their workout because it feels so great.

323.
The Thinking Thin like to look for ways
to get some physical activity into everyday routines.
For example, extending arm muscles when
throwing a towel over a high rack, squatting when
looking under the kitchen sink, bending from
the waist when hunting under
the bed for something . . .

324.
When they can't bear to bring themselves
to exercise, The Thinking Thin find that just
by doing a few stretches makes them feel great —
and often kicks in an exercise routine!

325.
The Thinking Thin know if they pump
their arms briskly when they walk, they can give
their upper bodies a bit of a workout too.

326.
The Thinking Thin know
not to try a gym program that's too advanced.
It will only discourage them.

327.
The Thinking Thin know almost no one is permanently fat.

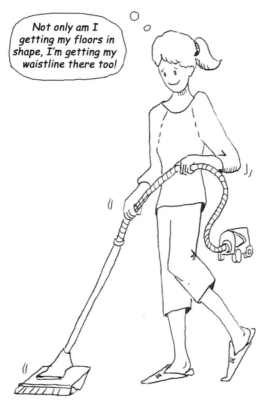

Not only am I getting my floors in shape, I'm getting my waistline there too!

328.
Sometimes The Thinking Thin enjoy doing chores because they know their bodies are keeping active.

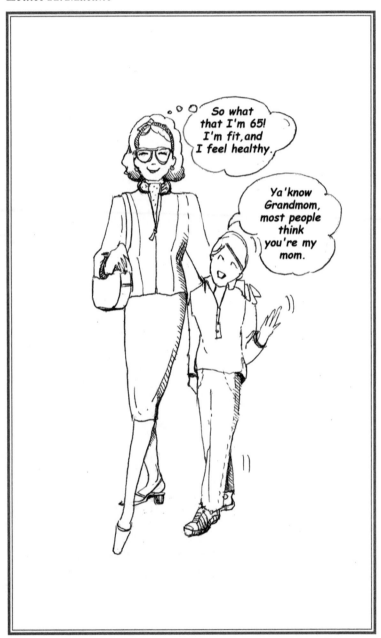

⚘

. . . *Their Health*

329.
The Thinking Thin understand
that if they indulge now — they pay later.
Their whole mind-set is to take personal
responsibility for their health where they can.

330.
The Thinking Thin believe it's not about their
numerical weight; it's about taking care of their heart,
their liver, their kidney, etc. with good nutrition.
These organs work hard to keep them healthy.
A weight-loss benefit is
a nice by-product.

331.
The Thinking Thin do not give all
the credit to their genes for their healthy bodies.
They know they have a way of thinking
that works to keep their weight
and health in check.

332.
The Thinking Thin have learned to like
their healthy, fit bodies more than indulging in
overeating. This is very empowering.

333.
The Thinking Thin find relaxing, by deep
breathing, is a good way to bust stress — and the
tendency to overeat that may go with that stress.

334.
The Thinking Thin listen to their bodies' needs.
If they feel sluggish, they know it's time to rev up
their circulation with some physical activity.

335.
The Thinking Thin know the good nutrients
in the food they eat enhance their eating experience.
Because along with good flavor, and satiation,
they know they are doing something good
for their bodies.

336.
The Thinking Thin incorporate lots of antioxidant
foods (like carrots and tomatoes) into their diets,
because they know these are great preventative
measures to certain diseases.

337.
The
Thinking Thin
are closet
"non-eaters."
When no one's
looking
they still
maintain their
good eating
habits.

338.
Whatever their weight,
The Thinking Thin aspire to be fit and toned.

339.
The Thinking Thin would rather feel better
about the healthy benefits of a nutritious food
than the taste sensation of an indulgent food.

340.
The Thinking Thin know they need lots
of hydration and they get that from unsweetened,
non-caffeine, non-alcoholic liquids.

341.
And they know they need protein
for muscle preservation.

342.
The Thinking Thin realize that sometimes their
bodies just want to hang on to every morsel they eat.
So they make wise choices in what they consume.

343.
The Thinking Thin believe the absence
of a personal trainer is no reason
to be out of shape.

344.
The Thinking Thin know that even with
all their good food choices they may not be getting
all their required nutrients, so they often supplement
their diet with a good multivitamin.

345.
The Thinking Thin believe their taste buds
prefer healthy foods because they've become
accustomed to them.

346.
The Thinking Thin know fruits and vegetables
are rich in antioxidant vitamins which can often
fend off environmental damage to the skin.

347.
Some Thinking Thin find leafy green
vegetables, beans, fish oils, nuts, and multigrain
breads may even help stave off wrinkles!

348.
The Thinking Thin realize constant
practice of these many learned eating skills creates
healthy habits that become next to natural.

349.
The Thinking Thin often look for cereals
and breads enriched with fiber. (Why get the plain
stuff when the fiber can benefit them?)

350.
The Thinking Thin know certain foods
work for them in additional ways. For example,
lean chicken meat has protein that gives them energy;
leafy greens have iron for strength (think Popeye);
and the vitamin C found in oranges
helps to fight off colds.

351.
The Thinking Thin do not want to hurt
their bodies with bad food.

352.
The Thinking Thin know their bodies
have to work unnecessarily hard to get back
into a balance if they overeat.

353.
The Thinking Thin know a little fat
on the body is necessary.

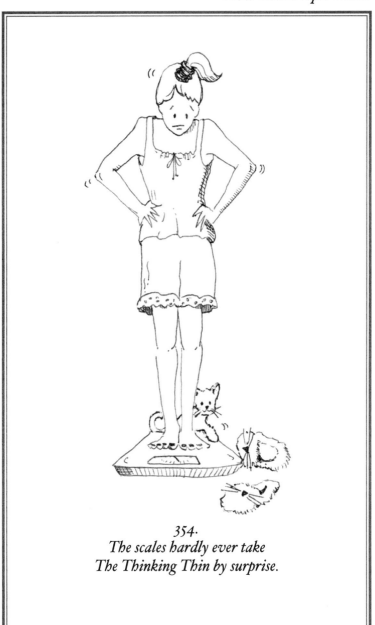

354.
The scales hardly ever take
The Thinking Thin by surprise.

355.
The
Thinking
Thin envision their
bodies as beautifully
functioning
machines
that have to be
fueled in an
optimal
way.

356.
The Thinking Thin know that some
people are healthy and their bodies are toned
and fit, even though most others would
not consider them "thin."

357.
The Thinking Thin realize that the last half
of the 20th century is probably the only time in human
existence that civilization actually paid to lose weight.
What an indication that food consumption
is out of control!

358.
The Thinking Thin know there is no reason
to panic or celebrate the gain or loss of a pound.
They know their bodies' weight fluctuates even over
the course of a day. It's not about what the scales say,
it's about an approach to nourishing their bodies.
Most bodies will adjust (in size)
to the right nourishment.

359.
Many of The Thinking Thin do not focus
that much on the "look" of their bodies. They focus
on healthy eating, some moderate exercise,
and occasional treats. An attractive body
is their reward for its proper care.

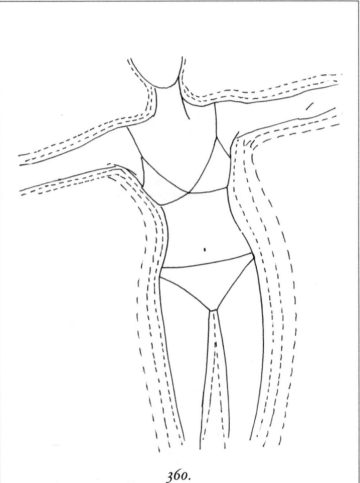

360.
The Thinking Thin know everyone
has a good body underneath any "bad habits."
(For those "who are not so happy with their weight,"
their best body is just temporarily hidden!)

❧

. . . *Themselves*

361.
*The Thinking Thin know it takes a while
to gain weight, so they are patient with the amount
of time it will take to lose it. That makes sense.
(And they are not so hard on themselves.)*

362.
*The Thinking Thin know
that to think like a victim is to blame something
out of their control for their weight dissatisfaction.
Weight is a controllable thing, unlike the plague
or the weather, birth origin, choice of parents,
height, ancestry . . .*

363.
*so they know it is up to them to be responsible for
they way they eat. They are empowered by this ability.*

364.
*The Thinking Thin find that eating with people
who think about food management the way they do
enforces their eating behavior.*

365.
The Thinking Thin do not blame
their genes for not fitting into their jeans.
(They know they ate too much
if their jeans are too tight.)

366.
The Thinking Thin slip up sometimes.

367.
The Thinking Thin know nature did not
give them a choice where fat is stored on the body.
They accept what they have and "work with it."

368.
The Thinking Thin bet other people probably
believe they can eat anything without thinking.
They can eat anything, but they THINK FIRST
about their choices and quantities.

369.
The Thinking Thin know not to compare
themselves to the models in fashion magazines.
Very few photos are not retouched.
(The waists are shaped, thighs slenderized,
and the skin tones evened out — no cellulite.)

370.
The Thinking Thin believe all people
are allowed to have mental gripes about
their body parts they dislike. But what they find
helpful is to just focus and be happy with the parts
they like. And everyone has good parts.
With proper nutrition and exercise their overall
appearance will inevitably improve and the parts
they dislike will most likely diminish
in importance.

371.
The Thinking Thin realize not
everyone's body has the same reaction to foods.
They find out what their specific food nemesis is.
(Pasta makes some people heavy; for others
it's dairy products, for example.) They learn
to minimize their intake of their "bad" foods
and increase their intake of "good" foods.

372.
The Thinking Thin keep in mind
that their children could be looking to them
as role models and they want to give them
something positive to aspire to.

373.
The Thinking Thin believe that just because
one is from a family of overweight people does
not mean one has to continue this tradition.
They know it's important to reevaluate
the eating habits they grew up with and make
better choices for themselves.

374.
If the Thinking Thin put on extra weight,
they realize it was their choice to select those foods
and eat those quantities. So they can choose to
lose weight -- by the foods they select and
their quantities! They are in control.

375.
The Thinking Thin realize that
all those models in magazines are just
that, "models." Models have certain
skeletal frames that make clothes look good.
The Thinking Thin have all different frames
and their primary goal is to be fit and healthy.

376.
The Thinking Thin know God gave them
a "casing" for the soul. It's up to them to maintain
and not abuse this gift.

377.
The
Thinking Thin
never go
on a diet . . .

but they
never go off
one either.

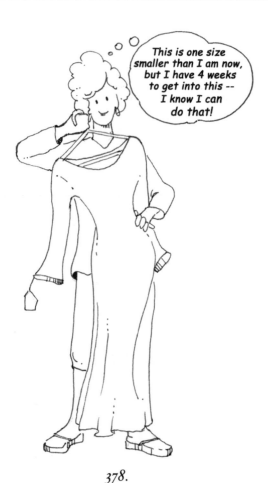

378.
*Sometimes The Thinking Thin buy
an outfit one size smaller for a special occasion
that's a few weeks away. This way they have
something to work toward — looking fabulous!
And at one size smaller, it's a realistic goal.*

. . . Clothes

379.
*The Thinking Thin work at making their bodies
fit into their clothes, not the other way around.
This is a little tougher than buying
new sizes, but well worth it.*

380.
*The Thinking Thin often use their jeans' fit
as an excellent barometer for keeping their
bodies in check.*

381.
*The Thinking Thin know the appeal
of the "Little Black Dress" is not so much
the dress — as what skin is revealed.*

382.
*The Thinking Thin know heels
will increase the ratio of height to width
on their body and make them appear*
taller and thinner.

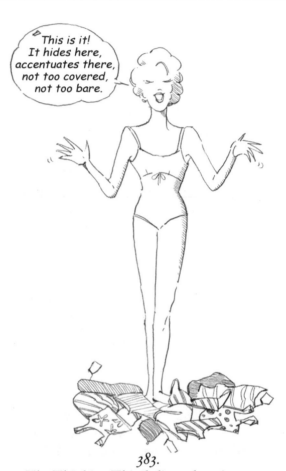

383.
*The Thinking Thin believe there is no way
any human being of the female gender should
ever spend less than an hour in the dressing room
looking for a swimsuit — with any fewer than ten
swimsuits to try on. And she should pay whatever
the heck they're asking for it! If it looks good on her,
it's well worth every penny for that confidence.*

384.
The Thinking Thin are not slaves to scales.
They know if they've gained weight by how
their clothes fit and how full they feel.
(Seeing a higher number than they expect could
merely be water weight that may disappear in a day.)

385.
The Thinking Thin know
nice shoes, manicured hands, and shiny hair
make for a great overall appearance,
but the major impression is between
the neck and the knees. (Ouch!)

386.
The Thinking Thin find that clothes with side
seams that curve in at the waist seem
to give the illusion of a waist that also curves in.

387.
The Thinking Thin do not put any significant
value judgment on what size clothing they fit into.
Dress sizes vary so much from manufacturer
to manufacturer. They forget what size
they're in, as long as it's flattering.

388.
The Thinking Thin know
the Americans' love of "comfortable" clothes
usually means manufacturers design to accommodate
expandable chests, waists, and hips. (This is a very
dangerous buying habit for weight control.)

389.
The Thinking Thin know to keep
trying on different styles and cuts and keep track
of which store or company brands fit them.
They know sizes vary too and find it helpful
to jot down the company or brand size
that fits them the best.

390.
The Thinking Thin often dress head to toe in
one color — an "optical illusion" to elongate the body.

391.
Even The Thinking Thin get
a "tummy" sometimes and know to avoid knits —
which often seem to accentuate any body flaws.
They feel better about wearing woven fabrics,
because they don't cling.

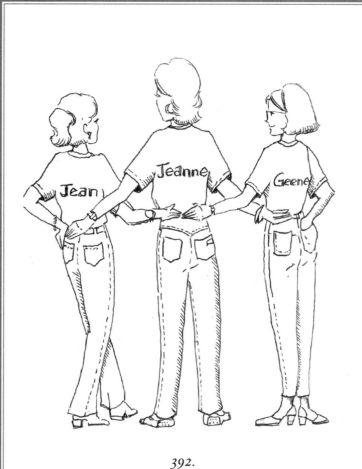

392.
The Thinking Thin know any company that brags it's the brand "that fits," does not take into account that people come in all shapes and sizes. Fits who? Even thin people can't all wear the same design or cut.

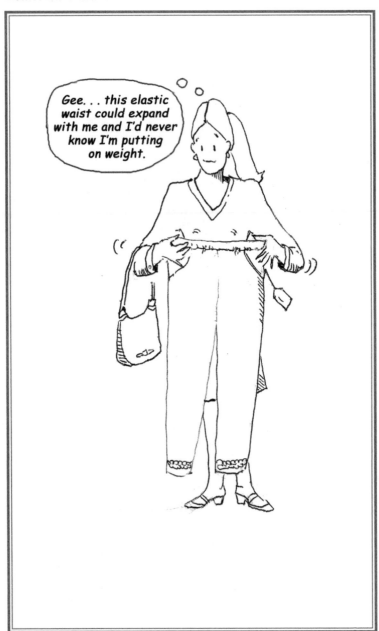

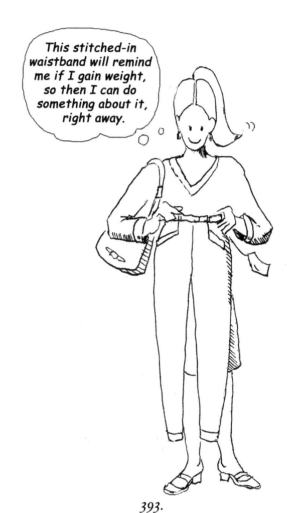

393.
Sometimes The Thinking Thin opt
for the stitched-in waistband. (This allows them
to keep a check on an expanding middle.)

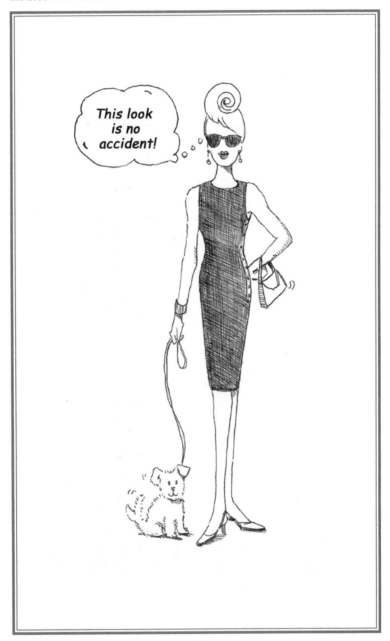

❧

. . . *Common Sense*

394.
The Thinking Thin base their
food management on common sense.

395.
The Thinking Thin know they have free will.
No one is making them destroy their bodies.

396.
The Thinking Thin do not get
swayed by fast-weight-loss tricks. They stick
to a regimen of sensible food management.
They have a "little" knowledge of the
nutritional value of most foods.

397.
Sur-feit: *sur'-fut*\\ *n:* excessive abundance *v:* to
feed or supply to the point of indulgence
The Thinking Thin try not to use the words
"surfeit" and "food" in the same sentence.

398.
The Thinking Thin think no one
should starve oneself to lose weight.

399.
A lot of The Thinking Thin are aware
of calories, but often they do not count them.
They rely on common sense.
(It's a good bet the chocolate Danish is higher
in calories than the whole wheat toast.)

400.
The Thinking Thin know if they stop
eating when their stomachs are less than filled,
there's a good chance they will not gain weight.

401.
The Thinking Thin know exercise can build
muscle definition, but if it's surrounded by fat,
they won't see much of that newly defined muscle.
They know they have to lose weight too.

402.
The Thinking Thin understand cause and effect.
"I eat too much —> I get fat."

403.
The Thinking Thin know food
is in abundance in the U.S. and it's up to
individuals to take responsibility for their intake.

404.
The Thinking Thin know that to gain weight —
they simply have to eat more than they burn off.
And to lose weight — they have to eat less
than they burn off.

405.
The Thinking Thin remind themselves
that their bodies are mostly water and they know
they need to drink a lot of it.

406.
The Thinking Thin know that if they gain weight,
THEY ARE EATING TOOOO MUCH
and their poor bodies have to stretch out
to store all that non-utilized food.

407.
The Thinking Thin understand moderation.
(OK, sometimes they trip up like anybody else,
but usually they practice this.)

408.
The Thinking Thin believe
their way of thinking helps reduce
many future health problems and lowers their
(and the nation's) medical costs.

409.
The Thinking Thin know babies need lots
of whole milk because it helps them to grow rapidly.
Adults do not need to grow rapidly.
They watch their whole milk consumption.

410.
A lot of The Thinking Thin believe
many popular actresses are way too thin.

411.
The Thinking Thin know anything
in excess can get them (and anyone) into trouble.

412.
The Thinking Thin know almost
anything they find fresh in the produce
department of their grocery store is nutritional.
And there are so many kinds of foods to try —
it makes staying healthy exciting.

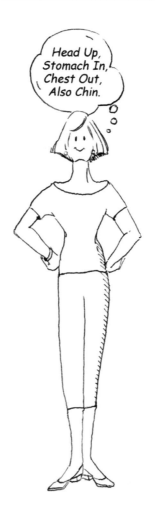

413.
The Thinking Thin know good posture
is the quickest way to look five pounds lighter.

414.
Beans are a low-fat source of good carbs and protein.
Since they come in so many varieties, they are an
excellent "food of choice" for The Thinking Thin.

415.
The Thinking Thin refrain from eating in motion.
This could lead to overdoing it, because eating is
not the primary activity. They would rather sit down
and eat, then they can focus on quality and quantity.
(And have a place to rest their food!)

416.
The Thinking Thin know if they cannot
lose weight, it's because they are not reducing their
food consumption and/or getting enough exercise.

417.
The Thinking Thin know everyone pretty
much has the same muscles and bone structure
that's on the standard doctor's charts . . .
they are just proportioned differently!

418.
The Thinking Thin know eating
is not a "free-for-all."

419.
The Thinking Thin know a crash diet
is a temporary fix and to change their bodies,
they have to change their attitude about food.

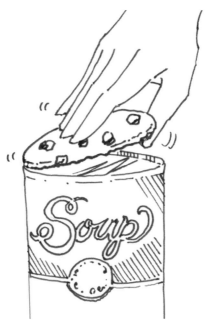

420.
The Thinking Thin find a "reasonable-size"
cookie should fit into the circumference
of the top of a standard soup can.
(Most cookies are made too big.)

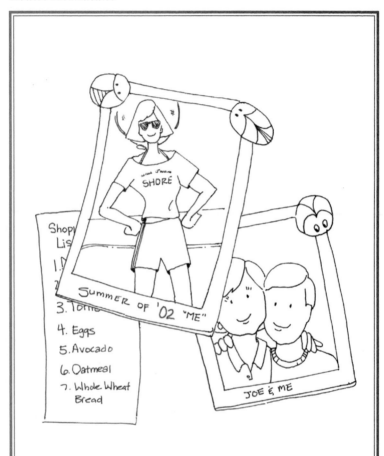

421.
*The Thinking Thin like to have a photo
of their "best body" readily visible. This reminds
them that there is this nice body underneath
any extra weight they might put on.*

. . . *Good Habits*

422.
*The Thinking Thin consider the long-term
consequences of bad eating habits and
the long-term rewards of good eating habits.*

423.
*The Thinking Thin believe a lot of those
"who are not so happy with their weight" have eating
habits that may go beyond satiation, into indulgence.*

424.
*The Thinking Thin try to eat three, square, modest-size
meals (and a couple of nutritional snacks) a day.*

425.
The Thinking Thin are not mindlessly munching!

426.
*The Thinking Thin find a small piece
of chocolate and a small glass of milk
make a nice dessert.*

427.
Many of The Thinking Thin split meals when
they dine out, especially when the entrées are very large.

428.
Since The Thinking Thin have learned to eat
more slowly, their satiation mechanism kicks in while
they're still chewing — as opposed to their gulping food,
and then realizing ten minutes later they are stuffed.
Then it's too late to monitor their eating.

429.
The Thinking Thin usually eat 21 meals
a week. They often designate one of those meals
as their "splurge" meal, and enjoy it without guilt.
One of these meals a week won't hurt.

430.
The Thinking Thin like to compare eating
to crossing a street. It's something they do every day.
But they do not mindlessly dart across the street.
They stop and look both ways. The same with eating.
The Thinking Thin do not eat without stopping
to think for a second if this is good for them.
There is a consequence, in both cases,
for not pausing to think.

431.
The Thinking Thin know it's managing
the little things that makes a big difference.

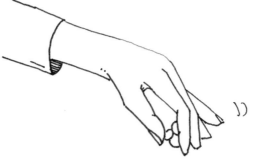

The right way to pick up peanuts.

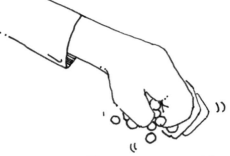

The wrong way to pick up peanuts.

432.
*When they have a bad day, The Thinking Thin
change their focus. (And they avoid making food
their instrument for change.) A walk is a good idea.
They know if they shift their environment,
they can often shift their mood.*

433.
*The Thinking Thin do not like to take the last piece.
(It looks like a courtesy but they're secretly thinking
"That's not going on my hips!")*

434.
*The Thinking Thin know pretzels are
a better munchy food than greasy potato chips.*

435.
*The Thinking Thin get "reasonable-size"
snacks at the movies (which in most cases
is always the small size). And they find it's a good
idea to get their friend to hold the snack food --
in the hand that's the farthest away from them!*

436.
*The Thinking Thin know everyone
is truly defined from the neck up.*

437.
The Thinking Thin consider smoking
a totally ridiculous way to control their appetite.
It is a crutch and an excuse for not monitoring
their own consumption.

438.
The Thinking Thin know it's important
to occasionally reevaluate their eating habits and
make adjustments when age or health dictates.

439.
The Thinking Thin refrain from the refrain
"I'll have another." If they listen to their bodies,
there is a good chance they are already
satiated after one serving.

440.
The Thinking Thin never suppress thoughts
of the foods they enjoy. They enjoy them all
(in small quantities, of course).

441.
The Thinking Thin try to make sure
their loved ones eat in a healthy way, so they
can help them lead long and healthy lives.

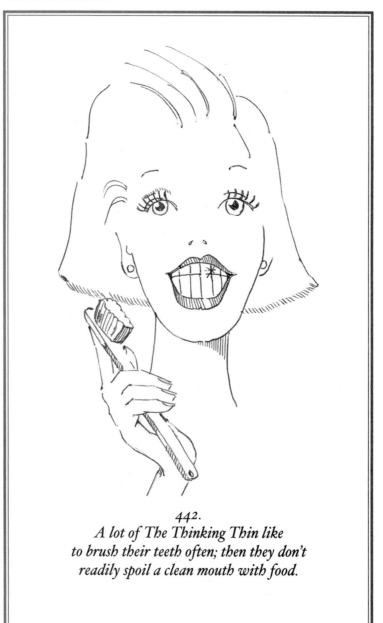

442.
A lot of The Thinking Thin like
to brush their teeth often; then they don't
readily spoil a clean mouth with food.

443.
Better yet, they floss. After all that elbow grease,
they're not likely to mess up their brilliant teeth
for a while. (And think how happy their dentists
will be — knowing they flossed!)

444.
The Thinking Thin know a lot, a lot, a lot
of water "flushes out" the system
and is a great help in managing weight.

445.
The Thinking Thin take all opportunities
to patronize their local farmers' stands. For the
urban types, it's the corner greengrocer.

446.
The Thinking Thin realize some people
give more thought to what they put into their
cars' gas tanks than into their bodies.

447.
The Thinking Thin "occasionally" order out.
This is a special eating event, and is not the norm.

448.
*The Thinking Thin know it's always wise
to enjoy a variety of foods in moderation. Even fats.*

449.
*The Thinking Thin believe
they've developed more finely tuned
taste buds because they don't overembellish
their food with sweeteners (which could
short-circuit their true hunger needs!).*

450.
*Some creative Thinking Thin sauté their food
in a little oil and a bit of water. This still cooks
the food well, but limits the oil absorption.*

451.
*The Thinking Thin anticipate big "event" meals
and often plan a whole week of food management
around this one big meal — then they enjoy!*

452.
*The Thinking Thin do not justify
"low-cal," "lite," or "diet" phrasing as
an excuse to eat a greater quantity.*

453.
The Thinking Thin like to put their food on plates and drinks in glasses, and avoid eating and drinking directly from bags, bottles, cartons, cans, and kegs.

3 Good Things to Do

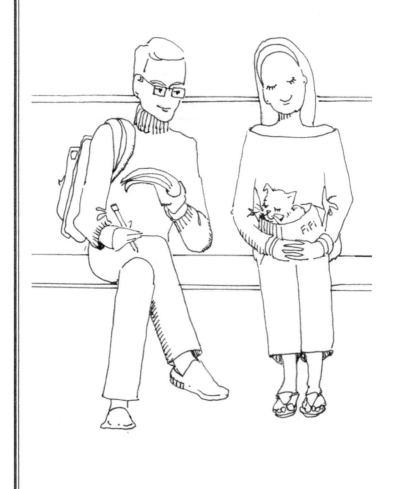

While Waiting, 1 Bad

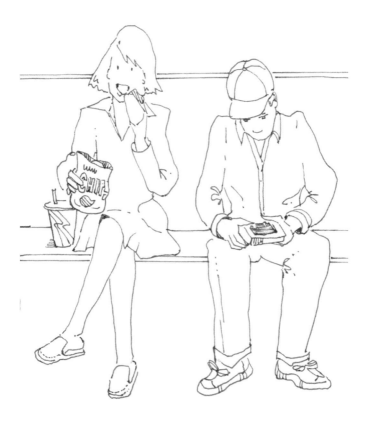

454.
The Thinking Thin realize there are
other things to do while waiting besides eating.

455.
*The Thinking Thin know it's a good habit
to grab a piece of fruit, along with their house keys,
before they head out the door.*

456.
*The Thinking Thin try to have only one hand
at a time holding a utensil while they eat.
(Except to cut food and swirl pasta.)
Two-fisted eating quickens consumption —
and it's rather barbaric looking!*

457.
*The Thinking Thin snack
on cold, crispy vegetables.*

458.
*The Thinking Thin know when
theyeattoofasttheirstomachshardlyhavetimetoalert
theirbrainstotelltheirmouthstoquitacceptingfood . . .
and that they are already satiated, thank you.*

459.
*The Thinking Thin know sitting up straight,
deep breathing, and stretching are three of
the simplest things they can do to feel good.*

460.
Some of The Thinking Thin
"shave" the butter off the top of the stick
for a very thin sliver. OK, it distorts the stick,
but better the butter, than their bodies.
(And it spreads more easily too!)

461.
A lot of The Thinking Thin keep a mental
check on their daily intake of the four food groups,
then they can compensate the next day
for any deficiencies. (No, icing is not
in the dairy group and french fries are not
in the vegetable hierarchy.)

462.
The Thinking Thin know any time
is the best time for someone to start thinking
as they do — the next meal is ideal!

463.
The Thinking Thin "choose" not to be fat,
by the foods they select to consume and
by the amount of physical activity
they build into each day.

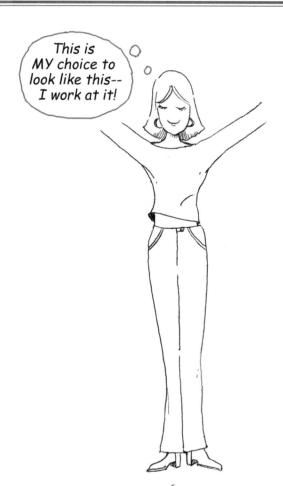

464.
To The Thinking Thin, eating is a very
important part of their day and they manage
each opportunity with the utmost responsibility
and respect for their bodies and their health.

Profile of the Author

Louise A. Masano has
spent over 20 years creating
commercials for major advertising agencies in New York.
Among them are campaigns for
Diet Coke, Revlon Cosmetics, Hyatt
Hotels, Brut Fragrance, Spring-
maid Sheets, and Snuggle Fabric
Softener, as well as for products to
help alleviate wrinkles, congestion,
and PMS. Six of those years were
devoted to creating commercials for
one of the world's most popular weight
loss products. From that experience,
along with her own distress of gaining
weight from "mindless munching," and then
subsequently losing that extra weight through
"conscious consumption," came insights
into how the ways of people who benefit
from a lifetime of thinness think and act
differ from that of those who constantly
struggle with food deprivation or resort
to diet gimmicks. In addition to
illustrating her book, Louise Masano
also enjoys portrait painting and the
piano. She lives
and works
in New
York
City.
☙

For additional copies please visit:
www.HowThinPeopleThink.com